AF616017

Preventing coronary heart disease

Coronary heart disease is the major cause of death in the UK, being responsible for 31 per cent of male deaths and for 24 per cent of female deaths in England and Wales in 1987. *Preventing Coronary Heart Disease* examines these statistics and focuses specifically on policies for its prevention by the government, general practitioners and concerned groups. Michael Calnan looks at the feasibility and effectiveness of these health policies and the obstacles in the way of their adoption.

Drawing mainly on the disciplines of politics, sociology and epidemiology, the author begins by examining the epidemiological case for prevention and then analyses what the British government is doing and can do. The government's policy is based on the role of primary care in prevention and the author discusses how this can be taken on board by GPs, concerned groups and the general public.

Coronary heart disease is of major concern to all those working in health and related industries, as well as to individuals. This book is the first study to look at the policies for prevention of the disease and will be invaluable reading for students of health studies and social policy, as well as professionals working in health care.

Michael Calnan is Reader in the Sociology of Health Studies at the University of Kent. He has published over 60 papers, articles and chapters in the area of health studies and is a national and international expert on policies for disease prevention.

Preventing coronary heart disease

Prospects, policies and politics

Michael Calnan

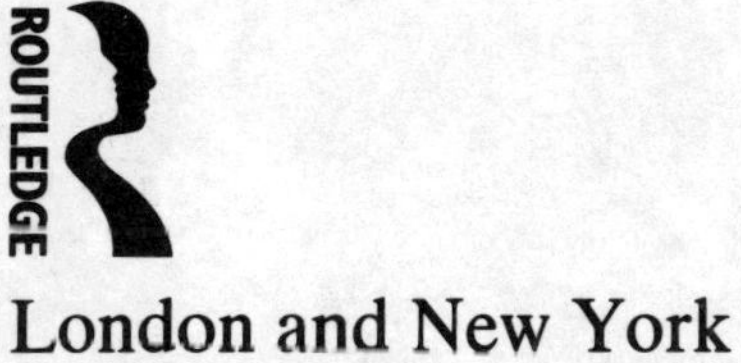

London and New York

First published 1991
by Routledge
11 New Fetter Lane, London EC4P 4EE

Simultaneously published in the USA and Canada
by Routledge
a division of Routledge, Chapman and Hall, Inc.
29 West 35th Street, New York, NY 10001

Typeset by Selectmove Ltd, London
Printed and bound in Great Britain by
Biddles Ltd, Guildford and King's Lynn

British Library Cataloguing in Publication Data
Calnan, Michael *1949–*
Preventing coronary heart disease: prospects, policies and politics.
1. Man. Heart. Coronary diseases. Prevention
I. Title
616.12305

Library of Congress Cataloging in Publication Data
Calnan, Michael.
Preventing coronary heart disease: prospects, policies and politics/Michael Calnan.
p. cm.
1. Coronary heart disease—Prevention—Government policy—Great Britain. [1. Coronary Disease—prevention & control—Great Britain. 2. Family Practice—Great Britain. 3. Health Behavior. 4. Health Policy—Great Britain.] I. Title.
[DNLM: WG 300 C164p]
RA645.C68C35 1990
362.1'96123'00941—dc20
DNLM/DLC
for Library of Congress 90–9140
CIP

ISBN 0–415–04490–1

Contents

Figures and tables

FIGURES

TABLES

Acknowledgements

This book would never have reached completion without the support of a number of organisations and individuals.

I would particularly like to thank the King's Fund Institute and the Department of Health for providing the financial support for the different phases of this project. A number of people provided valuable comments on the manuscript and I would particularly like to thank Mike Rayner from the Coronary Prevention Group and Ray Fitzpatrick. Thanks also go to the general practitioners who gave up their time to be interviewed. Finally, I am indebted to Jill Relton, Linda Steer and Jackie Newton for patiently typing the various drafts of the chapters. The views expressed in this book are solely those of the author.

1 [illegible]

The [illegible] of [illegible] practice [illegible] the [illegible] how [illegible] The [illegible] the [illegible] is [illegible] the [illegible] to [illegible] health [illegible] practice [illegible] crucial [illegible]

In [illegible] or [illegible] background [illegible] disease [illegible]

WHAT [illegible]

Coronary [illegible] (myocardial [illegible] arteries [illegible] details [illegible] arteries [illegible] these [illegible] this [illegible] which [illegible]

1 Prospects for prevention

The broad aim of this book is to examine policies for the prevention of coronary heart disease. More specifically, the book focuses on recent policy proposals which highlight the central role that general practitioners and their primary health care teams should play in the prevention of coronary heart disease. The following chapters focus on coronary heart disease prevention policies in general and how policies emphasising the role of general practitioners emerged. This is followed by a detailed examination of these policies and the assumptions that underlie them. Then, the empirical evidence is analysed particularly focusing on the feasibility of the proposals, the views of the general practitioners themselves and the barriers to involvement. The final chapter focuses on lay health beliefs and health practices and the factors which shape them. From the general practitioners' point of view an understanding of the lay perspective is crucial if their interventions are to be effective.

In this introductory chapter, however, the emphasis will be placed on setting the scene. Thus, this chapter will begin by providing some background information about the nature of CHD (coronary heart disease), the size of the problem and the prospects for prevention.

WHAT IS CHD?

Coronary heart disease is a condition where the heart muscle (myocardium) receives insufficient oxygen because the coronary arteries fail to maintain a sufficient supply of blood. (For full details see Open University (1985a).) There are two reasons why arteries cannot maintain an adequate supply of blood. One of these is coronary artery spasm (Bray and Ward, 1986) although this is usually a common accompaniment of coronary obstruction which is the major reason. Coronary obstruction develops when the arteries become more rigid and narrow due to the accumulation of fatty deposits (plaque). These fatty deposits are made up mainly of cholesterol and fibrin and when these deposits are prevalent the condition is called atherosclerosis (Open University, 1985b).

There is still some uncertainty about how these fatty deposits arise. Narrowing of the arteries is, in some respects, a natural product of ageing. However, there are more specific theories and two are popular at the moment (Open University, 1985b). The first suggests that fats move into the arterial wall from the blood where they help produce large amounts of scar tissue. The second suggests that blood clots that form the arterial wall are integrated into the wall where they degenerate into the fat and fibrin found in the deposits. The plaques themselves become the focal point for the formation of more blood clots which can sometimes completely block off an artery. In addition, a piece of plaque may break off and move down the artery until it blocks it. However, the main effect of atherosclerosis is to cause narrowing of the arteries and the severity of the condition is dependent on the location of these deposits.

How then does CHD affect people? It tends to affect people in three main ways by producing (Open University, 1985b):

(i) angina (chest pain) which can cause considerable debilitation. This occurs when cardiac activity is increased such as when an individual is exercising and the partial blockage in the arteries does not allow sufficient oxygen to reach the heart. This can cause cramp in the heart muscle which can be felt as pain in the chest or arm. The pain recedes once the exercise is stopped and the heart rate returns to normal.

(ii) myocardial infarction (heart attack) is where a part of the heart muscle is permanently damaged. This is where the coronary artery becomes completely blocked off and the deprivation of blood will lead to death of cells in the heart muscle. The effect of a dead patch of muscle in the heart depends on its extent and location. Sometimes it can lead to death although usually the person recovers. The pain of myocardial infarction is of a similar type to angina but it is usually more prolonged and severe and tends to be of quite sudden onset.

(iii) sudden death which is the result of the heart muscle suddenly stopping. This is usually due to thrombosis (blood clot) on a plaque.

SIZE OF THE PROBLEM OF CHD

Coronary heart disease was the major cause of death in England and Wales in 1987 for males and one of the major causes for females (OPCS, 1988). Thirty-one per cent of the total of 280,177 male deaths in that year and 24 per cent of the total of 286,817 female deaths were due to CHD. CHD also appears to be a major cause of premature death particularly in men. For example, CHD was the major cause of male death (34 per cent) in the age group 35–54 and in the age group 55–64 where it made up 39 per cent of all male deaths. For women the pattern was slightly different in that it was only the major cause of death in the age group 55 and above (OPCS, 1988).

There are also social class variations in the rates of mortality from CHD. For example, evidence from the Whitehall study (Marmot *et al.*, 1984) of 17,350 civil servants showed that compared with the highest grade (administrators), men in the lowest grade had 3 times the mortality rate from CHD. More recent figures for mortality in Great Britain also illustrate these variations by social class. For example, in between 1979 and 1983 for men aged 20 to 64 the rate of deaths from CHD per 1,000 population was 1.2 in professional occupations compared with 2.2 in semi-skilled occupations and 3.5 in skilled occupations (OPCS, 1986a). A similar pattern was found for women in that during the same period the proportional mortality rates from diseases of the circulatory system for women teachers was 76 compared with 111 for women cleaners and 114 for female assembly workers (OPCS, 1986a). Also, evidence from the British Regional Heart Study (Pocock *et al.*, 1987) showed that the prevalence rates of CHD at screening were higher in manual workers and the attack rate of major CHD events during follow-up was 44 per cent higher in manual workers.

The estimates for the incidence of CHD by age and sex for England and Wales, 1981–82, (Coronary Prevention Group (CPG), 1989) clearly illustrate how the incidence rises markedly in middle age for both men and women. For example for men aged 25–44 the incidence of myocardial infarction was 0.8 compared with 7.4 in the age group 45–64 and 12.8 in the age group 65–74. For women a similar trend was found in that the incidence of myocardial infarction was from 0.2 in the age groups 25–44, to 2.5 in the age groups 45–64 to 6.8 in the age groups 65–74. Data on incidence and prevalence of CHD for the male population rather than those who consult a general practitioner are available from the British Regional Heart Study (Shaper *et al.*, 1984a) which is a prospective study primarily investigating the geographical variations in the incidence of CHD. The study includes 7,765 men aged 40–59 years who were randomly selected from the age–sex registers of group general practices in 24 towns in England, Wales and Scotland. The prevalence of CHD was determined by an administered questionnaire and electrocardiography (ECG) to the 7,765 men in the sample. The data were collected at the beginning of the study between 1978 and 1980.

Data collected through the questionnaire showed eight per cent to have angina, nine per cent to have possible myocardial infarction and 14 per cent to have some kind of CHD which was angina or possible myocardial infarction or both. Evidence from the ECG showed around three per cent with major abnormalities and another 11 per cent with other abnormalities. There was some overlap between the reports in the questionnaire and the evidence from the ECG although over half of those with possible myocardial infarction combined with angina had no evidence on the ECG of CHD, and half of those with definite myocardial infarction on the ECG had no history of chest pain at any time. Overall, around one-quarter of the sample had some evidence of CHD on a questionnaire on chest pain or on ECG. This group was divided up into four per cent where there was evidence from the ECG and the questionnaire, ten per cent from the questionnaire only, and 11 per cent from the ECG only.

This evidence from the British Regional Heart Study suggests that CHD is common in middle-aged men in Great Britain. Further analysis of data from this study (Shaper *et al.*, 1984b) suggests that although CHD is common amongst this age group there is a low level of awareness amongst both doctors and patients. For example, only one-third of the men with possible myocardial infarction and half of those with a definite myocardial infarction on ECG could recall a diagnosis of CHD. Even in severe angina 40 per cent could not recall being told that they had heart disease. Overall, only one in five of those regarded as having CHD was able to recall such a diagnosis having been made by a doctor, and these were likely to be those most severely affected. This high level of unawareness amongst men about their own problems combined with similar unawareness by doctors of the true prevalence of disease and caution over applying the diagnostic label, is, according to the authors, one of the major reasons behind the lack of concerted action in this country to control CHD.

TRENDS IN NATIONAL AND INTERNATIONAL MORTALITY

High rates of mortality from CHD are seen as a specific characteristic of the twentieth century and a product of the social and economic changes brought about by industrial development. However, it is difficult, given the lack of detailed historical evidence (Bartley, 1985) to know how far the increase in prevalence is a real one and how far it is an artefact of changes in doctors' recognition or discovery of the disease. This debate remains unresolved although it does not so much apply to more recent changes in mortality where data are more reliable.

Deaths from CHD rose slowly both for men and women during the 1960s, and then in 1978 it started a steady decline up until 1987. Thus, in 1968 the death rates for men aged 35–74 was 583, by 1978 it had reached 615 and had decreased to 512 by 1987. This decline appears to have occurred in all age groups. The recent steady decline in mortality appears to be more marked for men than women. In 1968 the death rates for women aged 35–74 was 201, it rose to 207 by 1978 but had declined to 186 by 1987.

Internationally, the mortality rate for CHD (Shaper, 1986) in England and Wales has been described as being at a 'moderate' level. For example, in 1986 the death from CHD for men in England and Wales aged 35–74 was 439 compared with 701 in Northern Ireland, 623 in Scotland, 617 in Finland, 592 in Czechoslovakia, 590 in Ireland and 442 in Sweden. However, these figures are slightly misleading in that in Japan the death rate for that year and that age group was 67, it was 163 in France, 351 in Germany, 375 in the USA and 305 in Australia. Thus, England and Wales, while not at the top, are still quite high up the league table for deaths from CHD.

The recent steady decline in CHD mortality rates in England and Wales stands in marked contrast to countries like the United States and Finland, which between 1968 and 1986 have experienced a significant decline in mortality rates. However, it must be remembered that these two countries both had very high mortality rates originally, e.g. in 1968 both had male death rates from CHD of over 800. Perhaps the most dramatic decline has occurred in the United States. For example, during the period immediately after the war the USA experienced a progressive increase in mortality from CHD (Shaper, 1986). Since then, however, there has been a marked reversal in this upward trend (Epstein, 1984). Between 1968 and 1978 the mortality from CHD in terms of age-adjusted rates declined by 25 per cent for white men, 27 per cent for white women, 24 per cent for non-white men and 38 per cent for non-white women. The declines in each of these four groups have been markedly greater in younger rather than older age groups. In 1968 the CHD mortality rate in England and Wales was almost three-quarters of that in the USA. However, by 1985 the position had almost reversed and the mortality rates in the USA were around three-quarters of those in the UK.

This marked decline in the United States is claimed by some (Epstein, 1984) to be due in large part to the successful efforts of primary prevention, attributable in turn to improved eating habits, better control of blood pressure and a reduction in smoking. However, it is also accepted (Epstein, 1984) that another part of the decline will probably be explained by an improvement in prognosis and treatment. One explanation which has been neglected is what Pearson (1988) refers to as point source exposure and the decline in rates may involve the removal of this exposure. These exposures could be illnesses or social events such as depression or war.

In contrast, other countries' CHD mortality rates during the period 1968–78 (Pisa and Uemura, 1982; Thom *et al.*, 1985) have increased. The most notable increases have been in the Eastern European countries such as Poland, Yugoslavia and Rumania which have witnessed at least a 45 per cent increase during this period. Shaper (1986) suggests that increases reflect the increasing consumer demands for a 'Western diet' combined with an already high prevalence of obesity, hypertension and cigarette smoking.

In summary, CHD mortality rates in England and Wales are by current international standards at moderate levels whereas in Scotland and Northern Ireland they are high. Both countries have only very recently experienced a decline in mortality although this is only slight compared with the dramatic declines found in countries such as the USA and Finland.

There are also marked regional variations in death rates from CHD within England and Wales. For example, variations in rates in 1987 for men by Regional Health Authority (OPCS, 1988) suggest that the black spots for CHD are in Wales (422 per 100,000 pop.) and the North (446), particularly the North West region (441). Lower rates tend to be found in the Southern regions, particularly around the home counties (354 in the South East), in East Anglia (350) and in the West Country (359).

ECONOMIC AND SOCIAL COSTS

Elkan (1988) and Wells (1987) have estimated the economic costs imposed by CHD in England and Wales. Costs are divided into those which are the direct result of medical care and the indirect costs such as those stemming from absence due to sickness.

CHD in England and Wales in 1985 is estimated to have cost the National Health Service £389.9 million (Wells, 1987). The treatment absorbed one pound in every fifty spent by the NHS. The major part of the medical care costs are taken up with hospital inpatient care (£204 million) and primary care (£176.6 million). The remainder went on outpatient care (£9.3 million). Elkan (1988) in a similar analysis estimated the total direct costs of the impact of CHD as £431 million.

Wells (1982) also considered future trends in medical care costs and argued that because no dramatic changes in CHD mortality rates are expected in England and Wales at least in the short-term the shifts in the economic burden of CHD will depend upon the adoption of new forms of treatments. For example, it is estimated (Wells, 1982) that an increase in the operation rate from coronary bypass surgery to half the rate prevailing in the USA would cost an extra £26 million. This cost might be offset by savings on social security payments and increased tax contributions. For example, Wasfie and Brown (1981) have calculated that on average NHS costs per case of CABG are recovered within six years ten months as a result of reduced social security payments and the restoration of taxation contributions.

The indirect costs from CHD are more difficult to measure and to estimate. Certainly, the social and psychological consequences of CHD both for sufferers and their relatives are high. Levels of sickness absence are more easy to quantify and Elkan (1988) estimates that 34 million working days are lost per year because of CHD resulting in sickness benefit payments totalling £215 million. This excludes other social benefits that the sick may also be receiving. In addition, Wells (see Elkan, 1988) assessed the value of foregone production, due to absence from work, at £1,431 million at 1986 incomes. He also assessed the loss of production due to CHD deaths in 1985 at £2,412 million.

CONTROLLING CORONARY HEART DISEASE: TREATMENT

The evidence presented so far clearly shows that CHD is a major health problem in Great Britain. But what are the best ways of controlling it? This book focuses primarily on prevention although in this section treatment will be briefly considered.

The treatment of CHD is claimed (Open University, 1985a) to have three main objectives which are:

(i) The prevention of death immediately after a myocardial infarction
(ii) Prevention of disablement by severe angina
(iii) Prevention of further myocardial infarctions

It is clear from the above that these different objectives of treatment do not represent a 'cure' for CHD but are ways of relieving symptoms, improving quality of life and increasing survival.

Intensive care treatment (drugs and life-support systems) is used to prevent death immediately after a myocardial infarction although there is some doubt about its effectiveness. Rose (1975) suggested that only five per cent of patients benefit from being admitted to intensive care units as opposed to being cared for at home. There is the additional problem that most deaths occur within the first two hours after a myocardial infarction before it is usually possible to get someone into hospital. For example, it might be predicted that of 100 patients who had a heart attack (see Figure 1.1) 45 would die within a year and 25 of these deaths would be immediate.

The improvements in the treatment of CHD have mainly occurred in relation to the management of angina. Diagnosis of angina and decisions about the most appropriate form of treatment have been assisted by the development of a range of investigative techniques such as exercise testing and invasive investigations such as coronary angiography (Bray and Ward, 1986). One common method of treating angina is through drug therapy where the aim is to increase the blood flow to the heart or to decrease the work of the heart. There are three groups of drug which are currently used, sometimes in combination, for healing angina and they are (1) nitrates, (2) beta-blockers, (3) calcium antagonists (Bray and Ward, 1986). Surgery is the alternative method of treating angina. The form of treatment which has been the recent focus of a lot of interest and debate is coronary artery bypass grafting (CABG). CABG is a technique in which a blocked or narrowed section of a coronary artery is bypassed using part of a vein or artery from elsewhere in the patient's body. The objective of the treatment in addition to the relief of angina is the prolongation of life. The development of coronary angiography (X-ray examination of blood vessels) which allowed the precise identification of the size and extent of the disease paved the way for CABG (Bray and Ward, 1986).

There are marked variations in the operation rate for CABG within this country and between countries. For example, in 1982 the rate per million population (Wheatley, 1984) in the UK was 110 compared

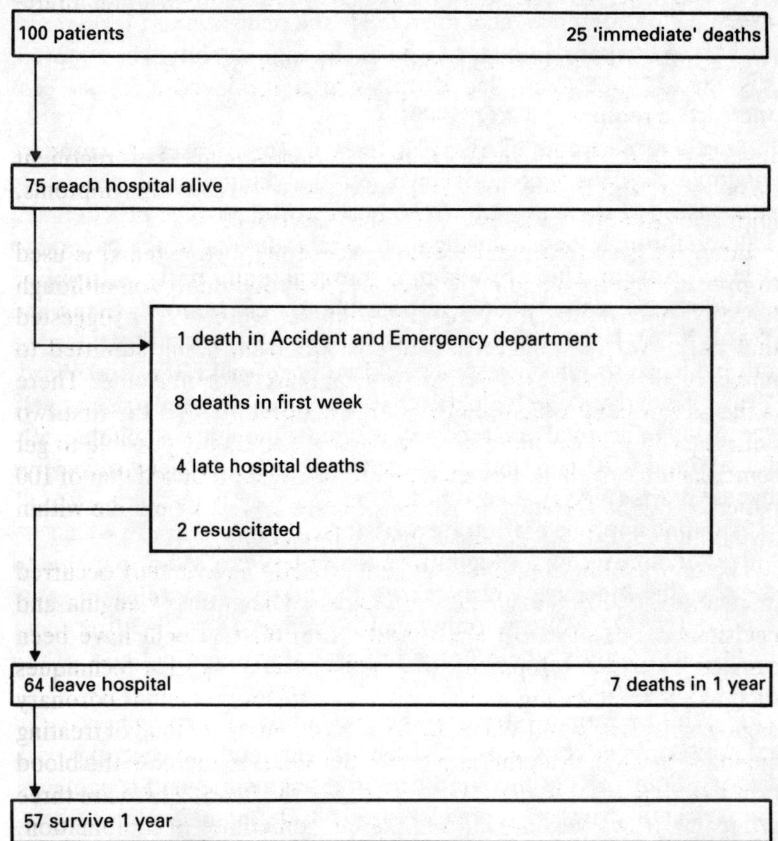

Figure 1.1 The prognosis of heart attacks
Source: Coronary Prevention Group (1989)

with 770 in the USA. The possible reasons for these variations have been discussed elsewhere (Aaron and Schwartz, 1984) but is it an effective procedure?

A series of clinical trials has been carried out to assess the value of CABG and the results from these trials were discussed at a recent consensus conference (King's Fund, 1985). This conference concluded that for the relief of angina CABG is effective in most cases where drugs are ineffective or unacceptable mainly because of side effects. However, for survival the situation is more complicated in that while surgery prolongs life in cases of severe disease there is uncertainty about its effectiveness in the treatment of less severe cases. The conference recommended that a realistic short-term target of 300 CABG per million for high benefit patients should be adopted. Figures for 1988 show that if this is to be achieved a 35 per cent increase is required (NAO, 1989).

One alternative to CABG, at least in some cases, is coronary angioplasty. This technique involves 'the dilatation of previously demonstrated coronary arterial stenosis by the passage of a deflated balloon through the narrowing then serial inflations of the balloon to a high pressure which results in compression and partial disruption of the atheromatous plaque responsible for the stenosis' (Bray and Ward, 1986). It is a technique which has been only recently developed but evidence so far suggests it could be beneficial (Bray and Ward, 1986). The advantage for patients is that it requires only a relatively short stay in hospital and recovery is rapid although it is suitable only for about 15–20 per cent of patients who might otherwise receive bypass grafts (NAO), 1989).

Another approach is intravenous thrombolytic therapy which involves administering a drug intravenously to heart attack patients to dissolve the blockage which caused the attack. According to some reports (NAO, 1989) mortality can be reduced by 20–30 per cent if this procedure is administered in hospital within 4–6 hours of the onset of symptoms.

The third treatment strategy, the prevention of further myocardial infarctions, involves the use of drugs, surgery and the control of risk factors. Some of the favoured drug treatments are anti-coagulants, anti-systemic drugs, anti-platelet agents and administration of beta-blocking drugs. There is still uncertainty about the effectiveness of many of these forms of drug treatment and, of the four groups, beta-blockers is the only one where there is clear evidence of benefits (Bray and Ward, 1986).

Attempts have been made recently to estimate the impact medical intervention has had on the decline in mortality from CHD in some countries. For example, Goldmann and Cook (1984) estimated that medical management accounted for some 40 per cent of the decline in the United States. In their analysis coronary care units accounted for 13.5 per cent of the decline, prehospital resuscitation accounted for 4 per cent, coronary artery surgery 3.5 per cent, medical treatment 10 per cent and treatment of hypertension 8.5 per cent. These authors note how crude these estimates are but suggest changes in lifestyle such as reductions in serum cholesterol (30 per cent) and smoking (24 per cent) have had a more significant effect. Similar estimates were found for the impact of medical management on the decline in New Zealand (Beaglehole, 1986) although a more recent study (Neutze and White, 1987) suggests that the estimates were too low and cardiac surgery accounted for 26–42 per cent of the reduction of CHD in New Zealand.

In summary, while there is evidence to show that some treatments for CHD are beneficial for certain categories of patient in terms of reduction in disability there is still considerable uncertainty about what impact some of the treatments have on reducing mortality. The evidence appears to suggest that the treatments may only have a limited impact and thus it may be necessary to look elsewhere at other methods of controlling CHD.

CONTROLLING CHD: PREVENTION

Before beginning the discussion about the evidence for a relationship between CHD and a number of potentially modifiable risk factors it is important to state briefly the terms on which the size of a risk factor is estimated. The commonly used method is estimating relative risk, i.e. how much greater a person's chances are of developing CHD relative to a person who does not live with that risk. For example, the relative risk of a fatal heart attack for a cigarette smoker is believed to be two to three times greater than for a non-smoker.

The other estimate of size of risk which is not commonly used but of equal importance is attributable risk, which is the excess risk associated with a factor in the whole population. The meaning and importance of using attributable risk in some contexts is illustrated by the following example (Rose, 1981) of the relationship between systolic blood pressure levels in men and risk of a CHD by age groups 30–39, 40–49, 50–59 and 60–69 years. The relative risk is seen to increase with increasing pressure and the relative mortality risk is slightly higher in the younger age groups compared with the age group 60–69 where the blood pressure gradient is slightly less steep. This is because higher blood pressures are more common in the older age groups than the younger age groups. However, being more common does not mean it is a good thing as when the attributable risk for this age group is considered the pattern is reversed. The absolute excess risk associated with raised pressure is far greater in the older men. The implication is that it is misleading sometimes only to estimate size of risk in terms of relative risk (Rose, 1981).

There is, as was indicated previously, still considerable uncertainty about the true causes of CHD. However, evidence from research has suggested that there are a number of factors which are associated with an increased risk of developing disease. The prevention of CHD is based on the possibilities of modifying these 'risk' factors and thus reducing morbidity and mortality from CHD.

Over 20 different factors (St George, 1983) have been identified in the literature by some commentators as being risk factors for CHD. However, there is some consensus about which risk factors are of importance. Some of these such as family history, age and gender cannot be the focus of prevention programmes as they are difficult to modify because they reflect biological differences or differences in genetic makeup. However, it might be argued that some of these differences, particularly the differences between gender, may be tied up with societal expectations about social roles which could be the focus of social policy.

RISK FACTORS FOR CHD

This discussion of modifiable risk factors for CHD will focus on an examination of a number of questions which have major implications for prevention programmes:

1 What modifiable risk factors are associated with an increased risk of CHD and which of these factors produce the greatest risks?
2 Are the associations between the risk factors and CHD causal?

Three potentially modifiable factors have been conventionally regarded as being of major importance and they are:

(i) cigarette smoking
(ii) elevated blood pressure
(iii) raised level of blood cholesterol (a type of fat)

Other factors which are believed to be of subsidiary importance are obesity, inactivity, diabetes, use of alcohol and stress although, compared with the first three, the effect of many of these risk factors on CHD remains uncertain or not proven.

Cigarette smoking

There is strong epidemiological evidence (Doll and Peto, 1976) to show that the greater the number of cigarettes currently smoked, the greater the risk of CHD. The risk of a fatal heart attack for a cigarette smoker is believed to be two to three times greater than for a non-smoker and it is greater in heavier smokers than those who smoke less. The relative risk from cigarette smoking (Doll and Peto, 1976) decreases with age. For example, at age under 45 years the relative risk of death in heavy cigarette smokers compared with non-smokers was 15 to 1 compared with a relative risk of 2 to 1 at 55–64 years. Doll and Peto (1976) estimate that for all ages cigarette smoking accounts for a quarter of deaths from CHD in people of working age (i.e. premature deaths).

Further evidence to support the view that smoking is causally associated with CHD comes from studies examining the impact of stopping smoking on the risks of CHD mortality. For example, Doll and Peto (1976) found that coronary deaths among male doctors aged 35–55 years who has been non-cigarette smokers for less than five years amounted to approximately half the number that would have been expected had this group continued to smoke. However, not all the evidence has supported this notion that the risk of CHD from cigarette smoking is reversible (Rose *et al.*, 1982). For example, recent evidence from the British Regional Heart Study (Cook *et al.*, 1986) shows that both current and ex-cigarette smokers had a risk of a major CHD event more than twice that in men who had never smoked cigarettes. Men who gave up smoking more than 20 years ago still had an increased risk. This excess risk among ex-smokers is only to a small extent explained by their higher blood pressure, serum total cholesterol and bodymass index.

There is still considerable uncertainty about the mechanism that links cigarette smoking and CHD. Carbon monoxide and nicotine have been identified as the most harmful chemical agents in smoking, although it has been suggested (Wilkinson, 1986) that of the two the more likely cause of excess deaths is carbon monoxide. The latter is believed to cause starvation of oxygen to the heart as well as thickening of the blood which can lead to a greater likelihood of clotting.

Blood pressure

There is also strong evidence to suggest that elevated blood pressure is a risk factor in CHD mortality. Evidence to support this association comes from a number of different studies (Reid *et al.*, 1976; Swales, 1981) although perhaps the strongest (given that the studies were well-designed) has come from two large-scale longitudinal (prospective) studies investigating risk factors in CHD mortality. The earliest of these was carried out in the United States and is called the Framingham Study (Kannell, 1975). This study monitored a sample of the population aged over 30 years throughout a period of 24 years. Both systolic and diastolic pressure was measured repeatedly during the study. Those taken at the beginning of the project were used to classify the outcomes for each individual. The major finding was that people in the study who had hypertension at the outset suffered considerable higher rates of CHD. The rate of CHD rose steadily with the level of pressure and the higher the pressure the greater the risk. This study also found that the people who developed hypertension usually had blood pressure toward the upper end of the range even as young adults. Most of these people were eventually diagnosed as having hypertension.

Examples of the relative risks are illustrated from the following figures taken from the Framingham Study. The results are based on systolic blood pressure which is taken when the heart is in contraction. The range usually runs from around 100mm Hg to over 160mm Hg. The latter level and above has been defined recently (US National Committee on Detection, Evaluation and Treatment of High Blood Pressure, 1986) as the level at which isolated systolic hypertension should be defined whereas 140–159 is described as 'borderline isolated systolic hypertension'. Below 140 is normal systolic blood pressure. Diastolic pressure on the other hand is when the heart is at the point of relaxation and has a smaller normal range running from 70 to over 115mm Hg. The latter level has been described as severe hypertension; 105–114 as moderate hypertension and 90–104 as mild hypertension. Below 90 is seen as normal although 85–89 is seen as high normal (US National Committee on Detection, Evaluation and Treatment of High Blood Pressure, 1986).

The results from the Framingham Study showed that for men aged 30–34 the number of cases for CHD per 1,000 population found in the category of systolic blood pressure <120 was 95; for the level 120–139 the number of cases was 157; for category 140–159 the number of cases was 243; for category 160–174 the number of cases was 265 and for the group 180 or more the number was 444. The overall rate of CHD per 1,000 population had increased in each level of blood pressure for the age group 50–59 although the overall pattern was similar to the younger age group. A similar pattern was found for women although the overall incidence was lower than for men.

The British Regional Heart Study (Shaper *et al.*, 1985), like the Framingham Study, is a prospective study although only focusing on middle-aged men. It is still in its prospective phase although results are being reported at various stages of follow-up. Recent results (Shaper *et al.*, 1985) have been reported at 4.2 years of follow-up and like the Framingham study, it showed that elevated blood pressure was a major risk factor. For systolic blood pressure there is an estimated doubling of risk for the top 40 per cent of men (i.e. systolic blood pressure>148mm Hg) but there is no evidence of any trend at lower levels. For diastolic blood pressure there is an estimated threefold increase in the risk of CHD in the top fifth (i.e. diastolic blood pressure >93mm Hg) relative to the bottom fifth (<72mm Hg) while the rest (72–92mm Hg) are an intermediate risk. Further analyses confirmed that elevated blood pressure was an independent risk factor for CHD as adjustment for other risk factors, pre-existing CHD and age made very little difference to the relative risks.

The evidence from these prospective studies suggests that high blood pressure is a precursor of CHD although there are doubts about whether the relationship is causal. The doubt about the causal relationship between high blood pressure and CHD arises out of evidence from studies which have examined the benefit of reducing people's blood pressure. High blood pressure is associated with obesity, heavy alcohol consumption (Shaper, 1986) and salt intake (Intersalt Co-operative Research Group, 1989). There is some evidence to show that by reducing any one of these or by treatment with drugs that there will be a reduction in blood pressure. However, the major question is whether lowering blood pressure leads to a reduction in CHD. There is some doubt about whether lowering blood pressure at the severe levels is of benefit in terms of a reduction in CHD mortality rates (Oliver, 1985) although at these levels the numbers of patients are relatively small. The more controversial issue is whether the treatment of mild hypertension is beneficial. The balance of evidence from the clinical trials in the USA, Australia and Norway (Truswell, 1985b) and in Britain (MRC, 1985) suggests that the treatment of mild hypertension is of value for reducing the incidence of strokes but little benefit for reducing CHD.

Why then is there such a strong relationship between elevated blood pressure and risk of CHD? It is possible that the relationship is not causal and the two variables are only associated with the link being a confounding factor which has yet to be discovered. For example, there is evidence that serum cholesterol concentration and hypertension are strongly interrelated as risk factors (Gotto, 1988). Alternatively, the relationship might be causal but the risk from elevated blood pressure might be irreversible. However, the view more commonly expressed is that there are major deficiencies in the trials. For example, the recently completed MRC trial of mild hypertension carried out in Britain (MRC, 1985) has been criticised for excluding a large proportion of 'high-risk' cases. The trials also tend to concentrate on diastolic blood pressure whereas systolic may be more important (Lichtenstein *et al.*, 1985) and easier to measure.

The actual mechanisms which explain the link between hypertension and CHD have yet to be identified. It has been suggested that the linings of the arteries are damaged by a continuous process of attrition (Wells, 1982) which might provide the basis for the development of artheroma. However, in the majority of cases (85 per cent) the causes are still unknown and this is referred to as 'essential hypertension' (WHO, 1983).

The incidence and prevalence of hypertension in Britain is difficult to estimate given the scarcity of comprehensive national data on this topic. However, according to Burt *et al.* (quoted in Wells, 1982) 30 per cent of the population has diastolic pressure in the range from 90–110mm Hg and 5 per cent exceeds 110mm Hg.

Blood pressure, as was suggested earlier, increases with age and thus many of the studies have concentrated in estimating levels of hypertension in middle age and older age groups. However, data recently published from a national birth cohort where the age of the men and women was 36 (Wadsworth *et al.*, 1985) showed that the prevalence of hypertension (>140) in men was 79 per 1,000 compared with 40 per 1,000 in women. However, although hypertension was almost twice as common in men than women, it was much more often unrecognised, and therefore probably underdiagnosed in men, and twice as many women as men reported receiving treatment. While hypertension is higher in men than women in younger age groups this difference is reversed after middle age when older women have high pressure (Swales, 1981).

Population studies have shown that elevation of blood pressure is associated with age, obesity, elevated pressure in blood relatives and race (Swales, 1981). This is in many respects borne out by the findings from an analysis of the national birth cohort data involving 36 year olds. The major predictors of high blood pressure in both men and women were fathers' death from hypertension and current body mass. Social characteristics were found to be of little significance after the other factors were allowed for.

Blood cholesterol

The third factor in the group of three major risk factors is elevated blood cholesterol and like high blood pressure there is still some uncertainty about its relationship to CHD. The basic hypothesis is that elevated total blood cholesterol or elevated LDL (low density lipoprotein) tends to be associated (some say causally) with an increased risk of CHD. However, elevated HDL cholesterol (high density lipoprotein) in the plasma is a protective factor (Truswell, 1985a). LDL and total cholesterol in turn are claimed to be influenced by diet with the major elevating effect coming from saturated fatty acids (Truswell, 1985a).

The discussion will then examine the following questions:

(i) Is there a strong association between elevated blood cholesterol and excess risk of CHD and is the relationship causal?
(ii) Does a reduction in intake of saturated fats lead to a reduction in cholesterol?
(iii) Does a reduction in intake of saturated fats lead to a reduction in the incidence of CHD?

No large-scale intervention trial has been carried out to answer all three different questions so evidence has to be taken from a number of different studies. Two recent epidemiological studies of cohorts of middle-aged men have shown that blood cholesterol is one of the major risk factors for CHD. The British Regional Heart Study (Shaper *et al.*, 1985) showed that, after 4.2 years of monitoring, there was a continuous and marked trend of increased risk of CHD as total cholesterol increases, e.g. men in the top fifth of total cholesterol have over three times the risk of men in the bottom fifth and men in the middle range have almost double the risk of men in the bottom fifth. A slightly reduced but still highly significant relationship between blood cholesterol and CHD was found after allowance was taken in the analysis for other risk factors, pre-existing CHD and age.

A similar pattern of evidence emerged from a study carried out in the USA (Martin *et al.*, 1986) involving analysis of 6-year mortality data for 361,662 men aged 35–37. These men were originally screened during a 2-year period beginning in 1973. The results of this analysis showed that CHD mortality increased progressively above the 20th percentile for serum cholesterol. The relative risk was large (3.8) in the men with cholesterol levels above the 85th percentile. It was interesting to note that for both CHD and total mortality the serum cholesterol was similar to diastolic blood pressure in the shape of the risk curve and in the size of the high-risk group.

There is still uncertainty, however, about whether blood cholesterol is causally associated with CHD although two major reports on the subject have given support to a causal link between the two. The COMA report (DHSS, 1984) on diet and cardiovascular disease stated:

> There is emerging evidence, requiring more evaluation, that reduction of plasma cholesterol in men may be associated with slower progression – or possible regression – of partly obscuring atherosclerotic lesions in femoral and coronary arteries.

The conclusions of a recent consensus conference (Consensus Conference, 1985) in the USA were less cautious and it was stated that not only is the relationship between the two causal but lowering elevated blood cholesterol levels will definitely reduce the risk of heart attacks due to CHD. Evidence to support this conclusion can be found in the results of a single-factor intervention trial known as the Lipid Research Clinic – coronary prevention trial (Lipid Research Clinic's Program, 1984). This trial compared the results of giving a sample of middle-aged men with an average serum cholesterol of 265 mml or above (top 5 per cent of the USA male population) a lipid-reducing drug, cholestyramine, plus a cholesterol-reducing diet, with those using the same diet together with a placebo. Seven years later at the end point of the trial the combination of diet and cholestyramine was successful in lowering the average plasma cholesterol level by 8.5 per cent compared with the placebo group and the prevalence of CHD was 19 per cent lower in the cholestyramine-treated group than in the placebo group. However, there was no difference in overall mortality between the two groups, suggesting that, coupled with a fall in CHD, there was an increase in mortality from other causes.

This evidence suggests that not only can serum cholesterol be decreased by a combination of drugs and diet but a decrease is significantly associated with a reduction in CHD. It suggests a causal link between serum cholesterol and CHD but does not provide an answer to the question about the benefits of dietary change for reducing serum cholesterol levels in the wider population. The trial did however suggest that dietary change can reduce serum cholesterol when levels are high. Mann (1987) came to a similar conclusion in his review of both primary prevention clinical trials and secondary prevention trials aimed at cholesterol lowering. Reporting an analysis of all the studies he showed that cholesterol lowering can, during a relatively short-time course, reduce CHD incidence so that a 10 per cent cholesterol reduction is associated with a 15–20 per cent reduction in total CHD incidence. While many of the trials have not shown a benefit in terms of reduction in total mortality the studies are of short-term duration and examination over a longer period should result in a significant improvement in overall mortality.

Evidence has been provided to answer the first two of the questions posed earlier but what about the evidence for a relationship between changes in diet and a reduction in CHD. Without a trial specifically examining the proposition it is necessary to turn to studies comparing patterns of dietary consumption and CHD mortality rates in a number of different countries. One such study (Keys *et al.*, 1981) compared average serum cholesterol levels of sixteen cohorts of men in seven countries with CHD rates over ten years. A strong correlation was found between these two factors and a strong correlation was also found between the average intake of saturated fatty acids and the coronary death rate. The authors concluded:

> The findings do not prove that saturates in the diet cause increased mortality but are consistent with the hypothesis that risk of early death is increased by dietary saturates in populations in which coronary disease is a major cause of death.

The picture is even more confused when data are examined which compare changes in fat consumption (Marmot, 1984) with changes in CHD mortality rates. For example, in Sweden there has been a decrease in fat consumption but an increase in CHD mortality and in Japan an increase in fat consumption and a decrease in CHD mortality. Thus, as Marmot (1984) points out, a single factor explanation will not fit all the observed trends and it is important to see CHD always as a Multi-Factorial disease. However, Shaper (1986) adopting the approach suggested by Marmot (1984) and also drawing on the evidence from the seven country study (Keys *et al.*, 1981) suggests that serum cholesterol and dietary considerations are of major importance and the influence of the other two risk factors are dependent on them.

Shaper (1986) argues that atherosclerosis of the coronary arteries is a necessary background for the vast majority of CHD events although it may not be a sufficient cause in itself. He argued that atherosclerosis and CHD have a fundamental nutritional basis. Populations with a high proportion of saturated fats in their diet tend to have average serum total cholesterol concentrations considerably higher than levels regarded as optimal. These populations are susceptible to atherosclerosis and CHD, and this susceptibility can be made clinically manifest by the presence of aggravating factors (risk factors) such as cigarette smoking and hypertension. Thus, in countries such as Britain and the USA where average serum total cholesterol is high, other risk factors, such as hypertension and cigarette smoking, are effective. However, in countries such as Japan where serum total cholesterol (TC) is relatively low but there is a high prevalence of hypertension and cigarette smoking there are low levels of CHD. According to this argument, the average serum total cholesterol in middle-aged men is a good indicator of a community's susceptibility to CHD. The population's diet determines levels of susceptibility in a country. Levels of saturated fats in the diet raise serum TC and levels of polyunsaturated fats lower it. The P:S ratio is the amount of polyunsaturated fats in the average adult diet to the amount of saturated fat in that diet. Internationally, the saturated fat intake varies much more than the polyunsaturated fat intake. As the ratio decreases from 1.0 (e.g. Japan) towards 0.2 (Great Britain) the incidence of atherosclerosis and average serum TC increases in severity and concentration. Thus, according to this approach the prevention of CHD should focus on nutritional action.

The claim that Britain has a relatively high average level of serum cholesterol is further supported by evidence from the British Regional Heart Study (Thelle *et al.*, 1983). The mean value for total cholesterol in this sample of middle-aged men was 242 mg/d which is higher than that observed in the USA at the time the article was written. There was little difference between two countries for the mean HDL-cholesterol concentration. The study also examined the relationship between concentrations of serum total cholesterol and age, social class, body mass index, cigarette smoking, alcohol intake and physical activity at work. Body mass was most strongly associated with serum cholesterol out of the factors. Serum total cholesterol increased with increasing body mass index until 28 kg/m2 but thereafter showed no further rise.

The difference between British blood cholesterol concentrations and concentrations in American populations (male populations) has raised doubts about the value of applying the recommendations of the consensus conference (Consensus Conference, 1985) to the British population (Shaper and Pocock, 1985). The consensus conference recommended that individuals with high risk cholesterol concentrations (above 90th percentile: >259mg/100ml) should be treated intensively by diet and if necessary be supplemented by drugs. Those at moderate risk (>240mg/100ml: 75th–90th percentile) should be treated with diet and only a small proportion would require drug treatment. Evidence from the British Regional Heart Study (Shaper and Pocock, 1985) shows that when the recommendations are applied to British middle-aged men 31 per cent would require dietary treatment coupled with drug treatment and another 18 per cent would require dietary treatment by itself. Thus, according to this evidence about half (49 per cent) of the male middle-aged population would require at the least skilled dietary advice and monitoring of blood cholesterol response coupled in some cases with drug therapy. A similar pattern of results emerged from studies carried out in Scotland (Tunstall-Pedoe *et al.*., 1989).

Shaper and Pocock (1985) also point out that the high risk approach of identifying those above the 80th percentile of the distribution of serum cholesterol for the population on which it is aimed to give advice may be more effective on the American male population than the British. For example, in Britain, using the 80th and 90th percentile would only identify 32 per cent and 18 per cent respectively of those middle-aged men likely to develop CHD. However, in the United States the comparable figures for the 80th and 90th percentile would be 49 per cent and 30 per cent respectively, suggesting that the population approach is perhaps the most effective strategy in countries with relatively high serum cholesterol concentrations.

A more recently published study (Mann *et al.*, 1988) found that mean cholesterol concentrations have changed little over the last decade or so. For example, in 1974 mean cholesterol concentrations of 5.8 and 5.9 mmol/1 were reported for men and women respectively in the age range 25–59. Twelve years later the comparable figures for men and women were 5.9 and 5.8. There was also a direct relationship between age and cholesterol level in that highest levels were found amongst the older age groups (55–59: 6.1 for men and 6.7 for women) and the lowest levels amongst the younger age groups (25–29: 5.2 for men and 5.1 for women).

MULTIPLE RISK FACTORS

Much of the empirical evidence described in the previous section focused on the independent effect of the three major risk factors on CHD mortality rates. However, in the latter part discussion focused on the fact that CHD was associated with multiple risk factors and these factors should not be treated in isolation from one another. There is some evidence to suggest that when they are combined, i.e. high risk on two or more, there is also an increased risk. For example, evidence from the USA Multiple Risk Factor Intervention Trial (Neaton *et al.*, 1984) shows that males' 5-year CHD death rates per 1,000 were 17.44 when the individual was a smoker, had diastolic blood pressure of >90 and blood cholesterol was >250. However, when the individual was a non-smoker, had a diastolic blood pressure of <90 and serum cholesterol level of <250 the rate was much lower at 2.40.

A similar analysis was carried out using data from the British Regional Heart Study (Shaper *et al.*, 1986). Using data on risk factors collected in 1978–80 from middle-aged men and examining the relationship between these risk factors and rate of CHD events by a 5-year follow-up the aim was to identify men at high risk of heart attacks. The factors included in the analysis were cigarette smoking, mean blood pressure, recall of CHD or diabetes mellitus diagnosed by a doctor, history of parental deaths from heart trouble, presence of angina, electrocardiographic evidence and serum total cholesterol concentrate. A risk score was developed based on these risk factors and the top fifth of the score distribution identified 59 per cent of CHD cases – that is, men who subsequently experienced major CHD events over the following five years.

Evidence from field trials evaluating the impact of attempts to change multiple risk factors on CHD mortality rates is mixed (McCormick and Skrabanek, 1988). There have been two different types of programme. One of these has involved the use of the approach called the 'medical model' which involves screening for high risk individuals. This approach aims to reduce the high risk faced by a small proportion of people here and now. A number of these multifactorial interventions have been carried out particularly in the United States (Winkelstein and Marmot, 1981). However, there are probably two which need to be described in some detail.

The first of these was carried out in Oslo, Norway (Hjermann, 1983) and focused only on changes in serum cholesterol and cigarette smoking amongst 'high risk' men aged 40–49. The intervention group received individual dietary and anti-smoking advice with visits to a hospital clinic every six months. The results indicated a successful change of both risk factors in the intervention group compared with the control, and the rate of fatal and non-fatal heart attacks was reduced by nearly half. The investigators attributed a quarter of the reduction in heart attacks to patients giving up smoking and more than half to falls in cholesterol.

The second of the trials was carried out in the USA and was called the Multiple Risk Factor Intervention Trial (Cutler *et al.*, 1985). This focused on high risk men aged 25–57. A 6-year randomised intervention programme was adopted with 50 per cent being allocated to their usual medical care source for management of their risk variables and the other 50 per cent were enrolled in special intervention programmes involving behavioural techniques for modifying changes in serum cholesterol levels and cigarette smoking behaviour and weight reduction and drug therapy for hypertension. After an average follow-up of period of seven years risk factor levels were reduced substantially more in the special intervention group than the usual medical care group. The differences between the randomised groups were stronger for cigarette smoking and blood pressure than for serum cholesterol and were achieved despite a greater than predicted change in the usual care group. There were no statistical differences between the two groups in CHD and total mortality. However, the mortality differences among non-hypertensive participants who resemble the cohort in the Oslo study of cholesterol and smoking intervention revealed benefits of special intervention compared with usual care. Although total mortality was not different CHD mortality was 35 per cent lower in the special intervention group. It is interesting to note that in these multiple risk interventions there appears to be clear evidence of reductions in CHD mortality rates only when hypertensives are excluded.

The alternative approach is the mass intervention programme which focuses on the population as a whole. It is more of a long-term policy aiming to reduce levels of risk factor in all members of the population. There are at least three studies which have used such an approach. One of these is known as the Stanford Heart Disease Prevention Programme (Farquhar *et al.*, 1977) where the aim was to see whether community health education could reduce the risk of CHD. No mortality data were collected as the study focused only on the impact of health education on changing risk factors. The risk factors under study were cigarette smoking, high plasma–cholesterol concentrations and high blood pressure. After a 2-year period, the risk of cardiovascular disease increased in the controls but there was a substantial and sustained decrease in risk in both treatment communities. The decrease in risk was similar in the two treatment communities suggesting that mass-media educational campaigning directed at entire communities may be very effective in reducing the risk of cardiovascular disease. The second mass intervention project, known as the North Karelia programme, aimed to change both risk factors and CHD morbidity and mortality rates (Puska *et al.*, 1983). Smoking, serum cholesterol levels and blood pressure were the major focus of the community programme. Changes in risk factors and morbidity and mortality in North Karelia were compared with a reference area and major population surveys were carried out in both areas at the outset (1972) and five (in 1977) and ten years (in 1982) later. The results of the 5-year evaluation show modest changes in risk factors and a modest decline in incidence of CHD was observed in North Karelia although it was more substantial in the middle-aged male group. However, overall mortality trends did not differ between the two areas over the 5-year period.

The 10-year results show that the net reductions in risk factors given in the first 5 years were maintained during the subsequent follow-up. Age-standardised CHD mortality among the middle-aged male population in North Karelia decreased by 24 per cent compared with 12 per cent in a similar age group in the national population overall. Most of the decrease in North Karelia took place after 1973. During this period (i.e. 1974–79), when the impact of the risk factor changes could appear, the reduction in CHD mortality was 22 per cent in North Karelia, 12 per cent in the reference area and 11 per cent in all Finland less North Karelia. CHD mortality decreased by 51 per cent among the middle-aged female population in 1969–79. This decline among women in North Karelia was also significantly greater than that in the rest of the country.

The third study was carried out in Europe and was called the WHO European Collaborative Groups' Multifactorial Trial in the Prevention of CHD (Borhani, 1985). It, too, used a community model of intervention and the results showed a reduction in levels of risk factors amongst the intervention group compared with the controls. However, unlike the North Karelia project, these changes in risk factors were not associated with any significant change in the incidence of CHD, at least compared with the control groups.

In summary, the evidence has suggested first that higher risks of CHD mortality are associated with combinations of the risk factors although each risk factor still has an effect independent of the other. Secondly, there is some, but perhaps not conclusive evidence, that reductions in multiple risk factors, either through screening or mass intervention, can reduce the incidence of CHD and mortality rates.

It is difficult to judge from the empirical evidence which, if any, of the three risk factors is the most powerful. The evidence described above suggested that it could be either cigarette smoking or blood cholesterol. Some have assumed that smoking is the major factor because the evidence for its causal relationship is more clear cut. Cigarette consumption is also easier to measure and collect data on than serum cholesterol and diet. However, as Shaper (1986) has suggested, there is some evidence to support the assertion that patterns of dietary intake in populations are the key to understanding the causation of CHD. This approach has been recently supported by Mann (1989) who argues that dietary change is the most consistent factor related to the change in coronary mortality, that the most effective dietary change may be a relative increase of polyunsaturated fat, and that the mechanism may not only work through lowering cholesterol levels.

SUBSIDIARY RISK FACTORS

The discussion above clearly illustrates the uncertainty surrounding the so called 'holy trinity' of risk factors. Not surprisingly, there is no less uncertainty about subsidiary risk factors. It must be remembered that risk factors are those that usually increase the risk of clinical CHD events whereas those that decrease the risk are called protective factors. It must be remembered also that the focus here is on modifiable factors so that although factors such as diabetes mellitus increase the risk, it is difficult to see how this factor can be modified.

Obesity

Although being overweight brings with it an increased risk of hypertension and hyperlipidaemia as well as an increased risk of diabetes mellitus there is little evidence to support the claim that obesity is an independent risk factor (Shaper *et al.*, 1985). An obese person in Great Britain without elevated blood pressure or raised serum TC will not necessarily have an increased risk of CHD. Thus, what matters, in terms of CHD, is not whether an individual is overweight, or obese, but how he or she became fat (Shaper, 1986). Obesity is the outcome of an imbalance between energy intake (diet) and energy expenditure (physical activity) and thus when considering body weight we may also be including the impact of another factor which is level of physical exercise.

Physical exercise

There is increasing evidence to suggest that level of physical exercise is associated with the incidence of CHD. However, only habitual vigorous sport or a high level of total energy expenditure (Morris, 1986), are consistently associated with substantially lower rates of CHD. There is also mounting evidence that such exercise is an independent protective factor against the disease rather than having an influence through body weight.

Two studies, in particular, have shown how levels of exercise influence the incidence of CHD. Paffenburger *et al.* (1978) in the USA observed that individuals not engaging in 'strenuous' sports activities were at a 38 per cent greater risk of first heart attack. Participants in vigorous exercise (e.g. swimming, tennis, jogging, etc.) were also found by Morris and colleagues (1980) in their 8-year monitoring of middle-aged civil servants to be associated with about 40–50 per cent lower risk of fatal heart attack and non-fatal coronary event.

The mechanisms underlying the protective effect of regular physical exercise are not yet firmly established, although it has been suggested recently (Morris, 1986) that it is aerobic capacity of stamina that is the element which is critical to health. Aerobic capacity may be defined as the level of exercise which can be sustained without the need for a significant contribution from anaerobic metabolism.

Alcohol

It has been suggested that the level of alcohol consumption can act as both a protective and risk factor in the development of CHD. The influence of alcohol intake on risk of CHD works through blood pressure. Heavy drinkers have higher blood pressures than light drinkers or abstainers (Truswell, 1985b). Systolic pressure is more affected than diastolic and the effect begins at about four drinks a day and shows a consistent linear trend above eight drinks a day.

The evidence to support the idea that light or moderate drinking is good for the heart is more difficult to find. Light/moderate alcohol consumption has been linked with lower blood pressures and lower risk of CHD and alcohol has been related to an increased HDL cholesterol concentration. This stands in contrast to smoking and inactivity which are associated with lowered HDL (Thelle *et al.*, 1983). However, as Shaper (1986) concludes, while there is no evidence that moderate drinking is harmful to the heart there is little evidence either that moderate drinking is beneficial. Certainly, the grouping together of teetotallers and ex-drinkers (given up due to ill-health) into the no-drinking category might explain why no difference in health status was found between this group and moderate drinkers.

Stress and other social factors

Studies examining public beliefs about CHD (Farrant and Russell, 1987; Calnan, 1987) clearly show that the public feels that stress is one of the major causes of CHD. Certainly, as Pollock (1988) argues, stress has increasingly come to be regarded as an integral part of everyday experiences. She argues that while much of the attractiveness of the stress theory derives from its seeming to reduce the arbitrariness of suffering, it also carries with it a significant sociological component. This can serve as a means of organising and expressing a variety of ideas about the social order relating for example to the issues of individual autonomy and responsibility, or to the ways in which society might be perceived as dangerous, repressive or pathogenic.

Scientific research into the possible link between stress and CHD, however, has only recently begun to develop which is surprising given the limited explanatory power of the traditional risk factors. The slow development of this particularly important area may reflect amongst other things the novelty of the concepts, the difficulty in measuring stress and the predominantly biomedical orientation of the studies. Certainly, the latter approach to prevention tends to place great emphasis on the need to change the behaviour of individuals and neglects possible changes in the social and physical environment.

The model of disease causality which attempts to explain the possible influence of stress on disease is called the model of general susceptibility. This model stands in contrast to the multiple-risk factor model which was the approach inherent in the discussion in the previous section in relation to the traditional risk factors. The latter model focuses on the individual and implies that the physical and biological causes of disease often work in concert with a variety of other causes, such as factors associated with an individual's lifestyle. The model of general susceptibility, on the other hand, examines why certain groups in the population such as unmarried people or socially and economically disadvantaged groups in the population have higher death rates than married people or more advantaged groups. One approach is to explain differences in susceptibility to disease in psychosomatic terms as arising from differences in exposure to stress. This is the approach which has been used in relation to CHD where recent approaches have attempted to develop models which focus on the role of social factors in the causation of specific diseases. It is an attempt to integrate the multiple-risk factor model with the general susceptibility model. In the case of CHD the conditions which are believed to generate stress are social and economic circumstances and life events.

Social and economic circumstances

The rise in mortality from CHD has continued among working-class men (Rose and Marmot, 1981) whereas amongst professional men the rate has changed little for the past 20 years. As a result it is now 26 per cent higher in social class V (unskilled occupations) compared with social class I professional occupations. The difference in women is larger which is mainly due to the reduction in deaths due to CHD in the wives of non-manual workers and increase amongst the wives of manual workers (Marmot and McDowall, 1986).

Evidence from the Whitehall study of 117,530 London civil servants aged between 40 and 64 has confirmed this social class gradient for men (Rose and Marmot, 1981; Marmot *et al.*., 1984). When men in the lowest employment grade were compared with those in the top (administrative) grade, the age-adjusted prevalence was 53 per cent higher for angina, 77 per cent higher for CHD type electrocardiographic abnormalities among men with angina. At follow-up, the 10-year coronary mortality was 3 times higher in the lowest grade compared with the top grade.

How can these social class differences be explained? The first explanation is that the traditional risk factors such as smoking, high blood pressure, obesity, inactivity and lower levels of glucose tolerance (Rose and Marmot, 1981) are more common in lower occupational social classes. Pocock *et al.* (1987), using data from the British Regional Heart Study, found that marked differences in cigarette smoking contributed substantially to the increased risk of CHD in manual workers, who also had higher levels of blood pressure, were more obese, and took much less physical activity in leisure time. The explanations for their greater frequency have been described elsewhere (Townsend and Davidson, 1982) although as Rose and Marmot (1981) point out these conventional risk factors only explain 40 per cent of the variance between employment grades. Also, a recent study (Morgan *et al.*, 1989) of changes in diet and coronary heart disease mortality among social classes in Great Britain suggested that recent social class trends in dietary fat intake are unlikely to account for the differential changes in CHD mortality.

These results suggest a need for a different explanation. One alternative explanation focuses on a possible relationship between job stress and the incidence of CHD. Karasek (1979) argues that job stress is influenced by two dimensions. One of these is the stresses associated with the working environment and the pressures associated with the actual work and the other is the ability of the individual to control the pressures. The latter dimension is associated with the latitude that individuals have in their work to manage the pressures according to their own requirements. Levels of job stress and job dissatisfaction are claimed to be more prevalent (Marmot, 1986) in lower occupation groups than higher.

There is still considerable uncertainly about what the actual mechanism is that might link job stress and CHD. Recent research has begun to indicate a possible link between job stress and blood clotting. For example, Markowe *et al.* (1985) found a difference in plasma fibrinogen concentration between occupational grades (low grade – higher fibrinogen) that was the order of magnitude that could distinguish between peoples who subsequently died of CHD and those who did not. It suggests that the lower grade men have a greater propensity to form blood clots and hence have a high coronary mortality. The second piece of evidence which emerged from this study showed that the level of job stress was significantly related to concentrations of fibrinogen and also made a substantial contribution in explaining the difference between grades of employment. It is possible, then, using these different strands of evidence to build a speculative model which suggests a possible explanation for a link between occupational social class and CHD mortality. This model might suggest that social class position determines levels of job stress which in turn influences propensity for blood clotting which in turn will influence the risk of having a CHD event.

Some authors (Marmot and Theorell, 1988) have suggested that there may be an interrelationship between working conditions and lifestyle factors which leads to an elevated risk of cardiovascular disease. Marmot and Theorell (1988) quote evidence which shows that occupations characterised as low on decision latitude have a higher proportion of cigarette smokers than other occupations. One explanation for such findings may be that boredom and lack of skill discretion may make the workers feel that they need to smoke in order to stay awake. Alternatively, in some occupations such as nursing it may have the social role of releasing tension.

A similar approach has been used to explain why there are particularly high rates of CHD amongst Asians living in Britain (Russell, 1986). Once again, it is argued that the traditional risk factors cannot adequately explain this variation and that explanations might look to examine the relationship between psychosocial factors and CHD.

Life events and social support

Another way stress has been linked to ill-health is through stressful life events such as loss of job, death of spouse, divorce or retirement. Some research examining the relationship between the first two of these (unemployment and bereavement) and excess risk of CHD has been carried out although no strong evidence of a link has been found. For example, according to a recent review of difference types of study (Cook, 1986) of the relationship between unemployment and CHD the evidence does not suggest that the physical health consequences of unemployment are specifically cardiovascular nor that the effect on cardiovascular mortality or morbidity is large.

A similar conclusion emerged from a study which examined the 'stress of bereavement' hypothesis in terms of its impact on rates of CHD. Jones (1986) using results from the OPCS longitudinal study described some of the main characteristics of the pattern and magnitude of mortality, principally from CHD, following widow(er)hood. The results of the study showed that CHD following widow(er)hood is less than 10 per cent in excess of that in all members of the cohort. A peak of all-cause mortality lasting for about six months after bereavement is seen in widows but in widowers the excess appears to be less sharp but visible over a more extended period. No such clear picture emerges for deaths from CHD. Jones (1986) concludes that the stress of bereavement hypothesis is not confirmed by the results relating to CHD deaths although patterns of deaths from other causes suggest it may have some value.

The fact that this study (Jones, 1986) has indicated an excess of all-cause mortality which is associated with bereavement suggests that there is something about human relationships which influences physical health and especially longevity. The availability of social support seems to have more of an influence on some groups than others (Berkmann and Seeman, 1986). For example, it has been shown that social isolation or lack of support is consistently associated with increased mortality risk among men. Certainly, there is a marked gender difference in CHD mortality rate although no evidence about the relationship between social ties and mortality risk from CHD is available at present. However, there are two basic questions about the possible relationship between social ties and mortality risk which need to be examined (Berkmann and Seeman, 1986) in empirical research. Both have implications for CHD. The first is how human relationships influence health or which relationships or what aspects of relationships are important or detrimental to well-being. The second is why they seem to carry greater mortality risks for some groups, e.g. men versus women.

In summary, the relationship between stressful events and circumstances and the development of CHD is potentially an important area of investigation although at present there is a lack of empirical evidence to assess its validity. The concept of chronic stress is important because it is a way of explaining the link between an individual's environment, including both social and economic circumstances, and his or her lifestyle and the development of coronary heart disease. Some writers (St George, 1983) have already made an attempt to try to integrate the psychosocial factors with the conventional risk factors in the development of a more holistic model of causality of CHD.

Type A personality and CHD

It has also been argued that certain types of personality are associated with a greater risk of disease. Coronary prone behaviour is said to be associated with a Type A personality which is characterised by a strong preoccupation with work and deadlines and an orientation that is ambitious, competitive, aggressive and impatient. Doubts have been expressed (Madge and Marmot, 1987) about both the conceptual and empirical validity of Type A behaviour. It is not clear what the social origins of the behaviour are or how it might result in disease. Some have suggested that it is also a culture-bound concept reflecting the perspective of the middle-class male. For example, Helman (1987) argues that the Type A individual is a figure of moral ambiguity, embodying many of the inherent contradictions in Western industrial society. In particular, his anti-social behaviour is rewarded in money or status by that same society. Helman suggests that the Type A personality should be regarded as a 'culture-bound syndrome' particularly of middle-aged, middle-class men, and one which condenses key concerns and behavioural norms of society. The empirical evidence is also limited. For example, Johnston *et al.* (1987) reporting on evidence from the British Regional Heart Study did not find any evidence to show that Type A behaviour predicts major CHD events in middle-aged men.

A THEORETICAL CASE FOR PREVENTION

The balance of evidence suggests that cigarette smoking, elevated serum cholesterol and high blood pressure are the major potentially modifiable risk factors for CHD with vigorous exercise acting as a subsidiary protective factor. Body weight and alcohol are important determinants of blood pressure but are not independent risk factors. Body weight, however, by its effect on the major risk factors can be used as an important indicator of risk of CHD. Stress and psychosocial factors have been implicated in the causation of CHD although there is still limited empirical evidence on which the propositions might be evaluated. Certainly, there is some doubt about whether the traditional risk factors can adequately explain the social class variations in incidence.

It must be emphasised that there is still considerable uncertainty about the causes of CHD and there is some doubt about the part that even the major risk factors such as blood pressure play in the development of the disease. However, this is a position which is not uncommon in medical and epidemiological research. Taking this uncertainty into account, the actual contribution the risk factors make to morbidity and mortality from CHD should not be over-exaggerated. A large number of patients with CHD do not have risk factors and the great majority of people with risk factors do not develop CHD. For example, Marmot and Winkelstein (1975) in their analysis of eight studies in the USA showed that if people with all three major risk factors are followed for ten years, only 14 per cent will develop CHD and if people with only one risk factor are examined only 5 per cent will develop CHD. Recent estimates (Open University, 1985a) suggest that if everyone stopped smoking and their blood cholesterol levels were reduced to less than 210mg per 100ml, then the mortality rate for CHD would fall by 8 per cent. If raised blood pressure could be avoided in future generations (given stronger evidence for the causal link with CHD) then the estimate might be increased to 20 per cent (Open University, 1985a).

The case for prevention of CHD is not an overwhelming one, at least, according to the present state of knowledge. However, the case for expensive medical technological intervention for CHD patients also has yet to be made and thus policies aimed at influencing risk factors may be equally, if not more, beneficial than those which focus on the provision of certain treatment services. Certainly, neither approach by itself will be the total answer and so the different approaches should be used to complement one another rather than act as substitutes. Thus, there is at least a theoretical case for prevention, and it is doubtful that such interventions cause too much harm although little is known about the psychological costs of screening (Stoate, 1989). Prevention is also believed to be relatively inexpensive although cost-effectiveness will be dealt with in the next section.

COST-EFFECTIVENESS

The assumption that prevention is necessarily cheaper than the provision of curative services at least in relation to coronary heart disease has been supported by evidence presented by Williams (1987). He calculated the relative costs per quality adjusted life year (QALY) of a range of different procedures aimed at controlling CHD. The QALY is an index designed to take account of the quality as well as the duration of survival in assessing the outcome of health care procedures. The procedures were ranked in terms of relative costs and the analysis shows that advice by GPs to stop smoking is an extremely cost-effective procedure. However, such methods of assessment have come under severe criticism from a number of different quarters. These criticisms have been well summarised by Smith (1987) who tends to focus on the theoretical and philosophical difficulties. Smith argues that in the quality adjusted life table there is a need for reciprocal commensurability between duration and quality of survival so that it is possible to say that there is nothing to choose between, for example, one year of life at 100 per cent quality and two years at 50 per cent. Smith suggests that to include some degree of reciprocal commensurability it is necessary to find out from individuals with health problems what they feel about a shortening of their present expectation of life as the price for a complete restoration of health if that were possible. Individuals would, if they wished to answer this question, need to know what expectation of life might be in their present condition and to be realistically aware of the nature and possible progression of the disorder. So as to obtain a general estimate, large samples of individuals with a range of defined conditions of impaired health, and an average value for each disorder might be questioned.

No such information is available as yet as the sets of quality ratings used in most studies are based on small samples of arbitrarily chosen respondents. In addition, the quality measures are limited to two dimensions categorising 'disability' and 'distress' and ignore some other dimensions such as inability to carry out activities of daily living, pain, fear, self-image, stigma, etc. Also, most studies have applied these ratings, not to the course of the illness of actual patient, but to a standard 'typical' course as judged by 'experts'.

The application of the QALY in this context is to assist decisions about which treatments are of most benefit to patients with a particular disease. This is according to Smith (1987) a legitimate way of using

QALYs. However, for Smith (1987), both methodological and moral questions are raised by applying QALYs to decisions about treatments for quite different diseases as this is essentially a resource allocation decision about which patients should be treated. The methodological difficulty is that to assess the comparative usefulness of treating different diseases or patients, one must calculate for each the difference in QALYs arising from treating and not treating the disorder, since what must be compared are the gains in QALYs. The moral difficulty is the fact that cost-effectiveness assessments tend to favour patients whose age or disease confers the prospect of longer and better quality survival. Old and very sick patients will be placed by resource allocation decisions in a position of double jeopardy.

Alternative approaches have been developed to assess the benefits of prevention programmes. For example, L.D. Russell (1986) 'in an economic analysis of blood pressure screening' suggests that the costs of the programme should include (i) the costs of the treatment itself, including drugs, visits to doctors, and lab tests; (ii) the cost of treating the side effects of the drugs; (iii) minus the saving in medical costs because disease is prevented; (iv) plus the cost of medical care in the years of life added by treatment. On the other hand, the health effects include the added years of life expected from treatment, plus improvements in health during years that would have been lived anyway minus any deterioration in health because of the side effects of treatment.

Some other studies, as Russell suggests, have cast doubt upon the assumption that prevention is a better choice than cure in every case. For example, one study (see L.D. Russell, 1986) compared a change in diet for 10-year-old boys whose cholesterol levels were high with a policy of no prevention and intensive care for the extra heart attacks. The results showed that the cost per year of life saved was somewhat less for the intensive care strategy. Another study (see L.D. Russell, 1986) compared the drug treatment of hypertension to prevent heart disease with bypass surgery for heart disease once it occurred. The results showed that the costs of screening and drug therapy for hypertension were about the same per year of life gained as the cost of bypass surgery for patients whose symptoms were obvious without screening tests. However, when compliance to the drug regimen was less than perfect, bypass surgery was more cost-effective.

In summary, while there is some evidence to say that a preventive programme for CHD is relatively cost-effective, the case once again is not overwhelming, particularly when all aspects of screening programmes are rigorously costed.

STRATEGIES FOR PREVENTION

The aim of the discussion in the previous section was to identify the risk factors which are strongly associated with CHD so that the subsequent discussion of policies for prevention could be grounded in firm epidemiological evidence. This brief review suggested that policies related to the control of smoking, diet and serum cholesterol, blood pressure and its determinants along with the encouragement of vigorous exercise should be, at the least, the major focus of any policy analysis. However, this concentration on 'lifestyle' as opposed to psychosocial factors does not mean that the policy debate will exclude a discussion of the various policy options associated with changes in the social and physical environment. Clearly, patterns of food consumption and cigarette consumption are influenced by social and economic circumstances and any policy discussion must take that into account. Also, lifestyle factors alone by no means account for the relationship between social and economic factors and CHD and the impact of socio-economic circumstances may have more of a direct impact on health rather than mediated through health-related behaviour.

This review focused on strategies for primary prevention. Primary prevention aims at removing the causative agents which in this case are the risk factors or the factor which might determine the risk factors. It is less concerned with secondary prevention which has the general aim of improving the results from therapy, partly by early detection or tertiary prevention, which covers the care directed at general support and alleviation of the problems associated with disease.

The discussion about the causal relationships between some risk factors and CHD highlighted some of the differences in approach to prevention advocated by epidemiologists. The two strategies which have been proposed on the basis of epidemiological evidence are the high-risk strategy and the mass strategy or the population approach. The latter approach has been termed the public health approach because the measures advocated focus on the population as a whole. The high-risk approach has been termed the 'medical' approach because it focuses on screening for individuals at high risk so that they can be 'treated' by drugs or given advice about changes in lifestyle.

The basic aim of the mass intervention approach is to endeavour to lower the whole distribution of the risk variable by some measure in which all participate. The approach is a long-term measure and its benefits will probably accrue to generations ahead. The epidemiological case for the mass intervention approach (Rose, 1981) is that large proportions of the deaths occur to those with slightly raised or moderate risk levels of hypertension or hyperlipidemia. Thus, however successful the high-risk strategy may be for individuals within the top 20th percentile it cannot influence the large proportion of deaths occurring among the many people with slightly raised blood pressure or serum cholesterol who have a lower risk. For example, most people develop CHD because moderately elevated risk factors are widespread. That is, more cases of CHD arise from the large part of the population in whom risk factor levels are moderately raised, than from the small proportion that are at extreme risk. Furthermore, the predictive power of the current methods of risk assessment is low, as shown by the distribution of serum cholesterol levels in subjects with and without CHD (Lewis *et al.*, 1986).

Others have suggested that the scientific basis is stronger for high-risk intervention. For example, Oliver (1985) argues because there is still low specificity of risk factors for CHD it is not surprising to find also that mass interventions aimed at populations who are at moderate risk such as the WHO trial of multiple risk factor interventions are of little benefit. Oliver (1985), drawing on evidence from the Oslo trial and the lipid trial, suggests that there is a better case for high-risk intervention although he admits that there are uncertainties particularly in intervening for those at high risk of severe hypertension. However, preferring screening to clinical case finding, Oliver (1985) suggests the need for screening for those above the 80th percentile of the distribution of serum cholesterol or blood pressure. He argues that there are three main reasons for this:

(i) specificity of risk factors is at its best at this level;
(ii) successful treatment of very high concentrations of serum cholesterol and of blood pressure require the use of drugs and this high risk should be acceptable to doctors who are concerned about the side effects of drugs;
(iii) ration of cost to benefit increases when intervention is below the 80th percentile.

More recent discussion about screening for cholesterol in Britain has highlighted many of the issues and problems in the debate about the relative value of the 'high risk' approach. In 1984 a consensus conference of experts from the United States agreed that cholesterol concentration in all American adults should be measured at least once. As we have shown, mass screening is only one type of population intervention. Should such a policy be adopted in this country? The answer to this question appears at the moment to be no and the consensus seems to recommend to test selectively for those who benefit most (Tunstall-Pedoe, 1989). There are many reasons for this support for selective testing. For example Smith *et al.* (1989) argue that screening for low level cholesterol does not satisfy some of the basic criteria for screening in that it is a test of poor sensitivity and specificity and availability of effective treatment for high-risk individuals is unsatisfactory. These authors conclude:

> screening programmes, in which doctors approach apparently healthy individuals to make them patients for a lifetime, ethically must ensure that treatment facilities are available, that treatment is of proved efficacy, and that it does more good than harm. These requirements have not yet been satisfied by cholesterol screening. Individuals with positive results would be alarmed and the others – in whom most coronary events will happen – would become complacent. In addition, there are not yet the services available to produce necessary backup to help reduce patients' risk of CHD without having to resort to drugs. Moreover, screening would be extremely expensive.
>
> (Smith *et al.*, 1989)

Others have been concerned that cholesterol testing should be seen as one part of a comprehensive, co-ordinated strategy to reduce coronary heart disease rate and not the only policy response.

There are also other problems with the treatment of high-risk patients by general practitioners particularly in the treatment of those with elevated blood pressure or serum cholesterol. For example, in the case of hypertension there are drugs which can be used to treat it and tend to be used if there is already evidence of CHD, cerebrovascular disease or the person is diabetic. However, drugs to control hypertension sometimes cause side effects, including impotence, tiredness, depression and shortness of breath but these can usually be avoided. Some doubts have been raised about the results of drugs to reduce mild hypertension and non-pharmacological methods are available. These include weight loss, reduction of salt intake, saturated fat reduction, change to a vegetarian diet and exercise and relaxation. While general practitioners may in theory be free to choose between the different methods in reality there is some pressure to adopt the pharmacological approach.

This issue had been recently raised in relation to the control of elevated blood cholesterol although a similar discussion took place a decade ago about the control of hypertension. In that case too the drug industry were actively supporting blood pressure screening and now they are supporting cholesterol testing. As one health campaigner put it bluntly 'If cholesterol screening takes off before backup, the drug companies will be laughing all the way to the bank' or as Vines (1989) puts it

> The worry is that overworked GPs have neither the time nor the expertise to give patients detailed advice about diet and exercise. Nor are GPs able to provide the practical support to help people to make substantial changes in their lifestyle. Without such backup, few people will have the knowledge or motivation to live more healthily. Most doctors concerned about their patients' cholesterol levels will probably adopt the time-honoured solution of prescribing drugs. Patients, too, may see cholesterol-lowering drugs as the easier option, and many people might end up taking them for the whole of their adult lives.

The drug industry have not been slow to capitalise on this market in that not only have they been devising drugs to treat elevated cholesterol but have also been spreading the 'word' about the benefits of widespread cholesterol screening. As Vines points out (1989):

> The medical press, often dependent on advertising from drug companies, carry frequent stories about the benefits of screening. Some medical organisations, such as the European Atherosclerosis Society, accept sponsorship from the pharmaceuticals industry. GPs receive most of their information from such sources, or directly from industry . . . In the US the importance of diet in lowering blood cholesterol was making the running 20 or 30 years before cholesterol-lowering drugs were available.

Little is known about the long-term safety of the range of drugs available to treat elevated blood cholesterol. Also it appears to be a very expensive approach in that some researchers estimate that the bill for drugs for only 5 per cent of British adults would come to £1 billion a year.

There is also the problem about lack of support and backup and many argue that it is inappropriate to carry out widespread cholesterol screening without adequate follow-up and treatment. Hence, the population approach or public health approach aimed at reducing everyone's risk is advocated. However, the problem is that the public health approach will only be funded by public money as industrial concerns will not eagerly promote a massive population campaign.

The debate about the relative benefits and costs of the two different approaches remains unresolved. However, rather than see them as substitutes for one another it may be more useful to see them as options which are complementary. The public health approach is concerned with long-term benefits where the high-risk approach focuses more on the short-term. However, it is evident that the two approaches have markedly different implications for policy, with the public health approach emphasising a central role for the government whereas the major actor in the high-risk approach would probably be the medical professional.

In some circumstances there is a specific reason for choosing between the public health and the high risk approaches. For example, the evidence suggested that while elevated blood pressure may be a strong risk factor there is some doubt about whether the effect is reversible. Therefore, the most appropriate strategy would be to try to prevent blood pressure becoming elevated in the first place and thus a public health strategy might be adopted which was aimed at controlling the determinants of elevated blood pressure.

These two different approaches have dominated the discussion about policy options in relation to the prevention of CHD. It must be emphasised that it is primarily a debate about different epidemiological approaches based on epidemiological and statistical evidence. However, it is limited in that prevention policies will be aimed at changing health-related behaviour or the factors that shape and constrain behaviour. The two approaches tell us little about behaviour. For example, why are there some groups of people who are at high-risk and what would prevent them becoming high-risk? Can the high-risk group be identified by individual characteristics such as genetic or psychological makeup or do they have social characteristics in common which explain why they smoke more, eat fatty food and tend to be overweight? An understanding of these processes might be just as useful for the development of intervention policies as restricting the high-risk approach to treatment. Alternatively, if the population approach is to be adopted it might be necessary to explain why the patterns of cigarette and dietary consumption in society as a whole exist as they do, as well as explaining variations amongst different social groups.

This chapter has attempted to set the scene by providing some background information about the nature of CHD, the size of the problem and the prospects for prevention. It is an area where there are still many controversies and uncertainties and where knowledge is constantly changing. The following chapters focus on the policies which have emerged over the last decade or so aimed at controlling CHD. The general practitioner and the primary health care team, as will be seen, appear to have a central position in these policies and as the evidence in this chapter has shown the general practitioner has considerable scope for playing a variety of different roles in CHD prevention programmes.

2 Policies for the prevention of CHD

The approach of government

The central theme of this book is to examine the role of the general practitioner in the prevention of CHD. However, to provide a comprehensive analysis it is necessary to look at policy in its broader context and that involves an analysis of the approach of the government. Current government policy, as we shall see, does emphasise the importance of general practitioner services although it is important to understand how and why this policy solution emerges and how it fits into other policy developments in the area.

POLICY ANALYSIS: UK GOVERNMENT POLICY PAST AND PRESENT

In the light of the evidence presented in the previous chapter, this chapter will particularly focus on the controls over smoking, dietary factors related to blood cholesterol, blood pressure and its determinants and exercise. The analysis will attempt to answer a range of questions which include what sort of strategy has been adopted, e.g. education, pricing, provision of services, regulation; is it effective in terms of intermediate outcomes such as changes in smoking and long-term outcomes such as changes in morbidity and mortality and the more difficult question about why it has taken the shape it has, i.e. what forces have influenced its development?

The second part of the analysis focuses on what could or should be done and draws on the evidence from other countries where alternative policies have been shown to be feasible and/or effective. So as to get a clearer idea of what shape UK government policy has taken it might be useful to draw on two frameworks which describe the possible options. First, the work of Sanderson and Winkler (1983) is considered which describes alternative strategies available to government and other agencies. Their work specifically applies to nutrition although it could equally be applied to the control of other substances such as tobacco and alcohol. They outline five possible strategies, which are:

(i) An education strategy aiming to induce people to change their behaviour through the provision of information, exhortation and instruction;
(ii) A substitution strategy aiming to encourage use of other commodities in place of harmful ones;
(iii) A pricing strategy aiming either to induce reduction in consumption of harmful substances by increasing prices or induce switching from harmful to healthy commodities by altering their relative prices;
(iv) A provision strategy aiming to change consumption directly by controlling the harmful products in government run institutions;
(v) A regulatory strategy aimed at controlling the production, promotion and availability of harmful products through legislation and/or administrative control.

Some of these strategies, as we shall see, have been adopted by the UK government and others have been rejected. The second framework put forward by Beattie (1991) (see Figure 2.1) considers health promotion more broadly. He distinguishes between policies which are prescriptive and come from authoritative and expert bodies (top-down policies) and those which are derived from or negotiated with lay people. The other domain on which he analyses health promotion strategies is whether these policies focus on the individual or are more collective or population oriented. Certainly, this is a useful way of analysing the focus of government intervention, although inevitably much of government policy will be prescriptive based on expert knowledge. However, the government does have the option of funding community health development programmes or of supporting the provision and spread of personal counselling by professionals.

UK government policy in relation to the prevention of coronary heart disease has taken two distinct forms. There have been those policy documents which have specifically focused on the prevention of CHD and recommended policy measures to control one or a number of risk factors. The second approach has been broader and rather than concentrating specifically on CHD has focused on diseases in general or one specific topic such as smoking or diet and health.

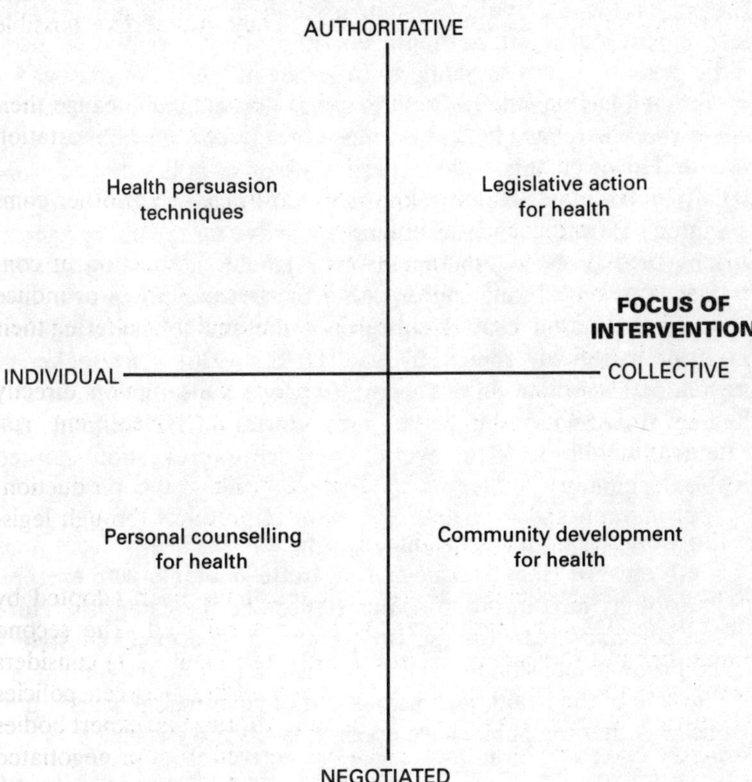

Figure 2.1 Strategies of health promotion
Source: Beattie (1991)

Clearly, these broader policy documents have major implications for the prevention of CHD and in many of them specific reference has been made to CHD. It is difficult to make a distinction between the two different approaches in an analysis of policy particularly as the policy measures recommended in the documents focusing on CHD only also tend to deal with controls on individual risk factor separately. This is, in some respects, not surprising given that different risk factors require markedly different options for policy. Thus, the main approach adopted here will focus on individual risk factors with the major emphasis on analysis of policy in relation to smoking, food and alcohol consumption.

THE CONTROL OF CIGARETTE SMOKING

The major focus of policy documents and initiatives prepared by government and its supporting agencies up until recently has been in the general area of smoking control. One of the major reasons for this is that it has been the only major risk factor, at least until recently, where there is relatively firm evidence of a strong relationship with disease. However, this is only a partial reason as policy decisions are not always based on 'scientific' knowledge and usually are made under conditions of 'uncertainty'. Smoking did arrive on the policy agenda as a 'medical' problem although mainly related to its consequence for the development of lung cancer rather than coronary heart disease. Certainly, it was a central concern of the first policy document produced by the government in 1976 (DHSS, 1976) which looked at prevention as a whole. In this report there was a specific reference to the important relationship between smoking and CHD although this statement will illustrate the overall approach to prevention adopted by this document:

> Probably the most important single factor which men from their youth onwards should ponder is cigarette smoking, with exercise and obesity next in order of importance. To the extent therefore that coronary heart disease is determined by a man's lifestyle – the prime responsibility for his own health falls on the individual. The role of the health professions and of government is limited to ensuring that the public have access to such knowledge.

Prior to that document there had been government activity in the area of prevention although much of it had been confined to smoking. Government policy in this area can take many forms, ranging from active intervention through legislation to passive support of the status quo. It might be argued that both prior to and since the 1976 document the government has adopted an education, a pricing and a regulatory strategy, although the overall approach has been piecemeal.

Legislation

There has been a limited number of major legislative measures adopted by the British government and doubts have been raised about their effectiveness. First, there have been attempts to control availability of cigarettes to under-16-year-olds. This legislation was originally enacted in 1933, but has been recently strengthened (Protection of Children [Tobacco] Act 1986) as a result of evidence from surveys which have shown that the vast majority of tobacconists (90 per cent) were selling cigarettes to under-age children. The second piece of legislation involved the banning of advertising of cigarettes on TV which was enacted in 1965 and was extended to commercial radio. Doubts have been expressed, too, about its effectiveness and in fact a recent survey of smoking behaviour showed that 23 per cent of smokers and 44 per cent of non-smokers still claimed to see cigarette advertising on TV (Marsh, 1984). Player (1986) estimates that in 1984 there were 330 hours of sport on TV featuring events sponsored by the tobacco companies and a survey carried out in 1983 showed 70 per cent of children claimed to have seen these advertisements. A more detailed examination of the way the Sports Sponsorship Agreement has been breached is shown in a report prepared by the North Western RHA (Roberts, 1986).

The form of regulation which is favoured by the British government in this area and others is self-regulation or more specifically voluntary agreements between the government and the tobacco industry. Over the last 16 years there has been a series of voluntary agreements. The agreements have been used for two different policies. The first of these is part of the government's safer cigarette policy through the publication of the tar and nicotine content of different brands of cigarettes, the phasing out of advertising of high tar cigarettes and the reduction of tar yield. This safer cigarette policy has tended to concentrate on lowering tar yields which may be important for other diseases such as lung cancer but not for CHD. More important for the latter is lowering carbon monoxide levels.

The second type of policy associated with the voluntary agreements has concentrated on attempting to control tobacco advertising and promotion. The agreements have concentrated on controlling tobacco advertising such as publication of the government health warning on cigarette packs and advertisements, cuts in cigarette poster advertising and restrictions on cigarette promotion aimed at young people. There have been voluntary agreements also in an attempt to control advertising at sporting events.

On the whole this series of voluntary agreements between government and industry has involved progressively tougher controls. However, claims have been made (Wilkinson, 1986) that these agreements or the spirit of them have been broken on a number of occasions and also that the voluntary agreements have been actually beneficial to the tobacco industry – e.g. they censure the continued allocation of a disproportionate amount of advertising to brands in the lowest tar groups (Cox, 1984).

Two new agreements have been recently negotiated. One of these was a new agreement to govern the advertising/promotion of tobacco products, and health warnings which ran from 1 April 1986 until 31 October 1989. The agreement included a range of different proposals including adoption of six new health warnings to be used on cigarette packs, posters and advertisements such as 'Smoking can cause heart disease'.

Other proposals included in the agreement have been documented elsewhere (Wilkinson, 1986) but perhaps the most important one was the setting up of a monitoring committee representing government and the tobacco industry in equal numbers. The functions of the committee are first to consider complaints about breaches of the agreement and secondly to appoint consultants to investigate aspects of the operation of the agreement.

The other agreement which was recently re-negotiated was on sports sponsorship and ran from January 1987 to October 1989. It too was monitored by the committee set up in 1986. The aim of the agreement was to tighten up controls over advertising at sponsored events particularly where the majority of participants were under 18 years of age although it was noticeable that house or brand names were still allowed to be used as part of the name of the activities.

Interestingly, while Britain has agreed to the adoption of health warnings, albeit on a voluntary basis, in its own country it has vehemently tried to restrict the European plan to strengthen the health warning on tobacco packaging (Raw, 1989). Raw argues that this resistance was a reflection of the government's opposition to the prevention of smoking and that these tough new warnings would not have been accepted by the industry if the British government had proposed them at home.

Fiscal policy (taxation)

It is only in the last six or seven years that increases in taxation have been used as a health policy measure for controlling smoking. The major purpose of increasing taxation before then was to collect larger amounts of revenue. This is clearly illustrated in the comparison (Calnan, 1984) between the typical retail selling price of standard tipped cigarettes and the retail price index between 1964 and 1980. Only on three occasions did the retail selling price of cigarettes go above the retail price index during this period. Any public health policy would involve at least the maintenance of the real price of tobacco, and prices during this period are believed to have fallen (Townsend, 1987) by over 30 per cent in real terms.

During the 1980s the situation changed and tax increases raised the price of cigarettes by 26 per cent in real terms (Townsend, 1987). The budgets of 1985 and 1986 further increased the price of cigarettes and the increases were well above the inflation rate. Townsend (1987) estimates that during the period of 1980–84 the increase in tax on cigarettes led to an increase in revenue of 10 per cent providing an extra £435 million.

The government has also adopted two other strategies for attempting to control cigarettes although neither directly involve the government. The first of these is the allocation of resources to the Health Education Council (HEC) to carry out a series of campaigns in the mass media informing the public about the dangers of smoking. The earlier campaign attempted to make the general public aware of the dangers of smoking. Lately, the campaigns have shifted towards attempting to change the social climate of opinion about smoking by emphasising the anti-social nature of smoking behaviour. The target group also shifted from the general public as a whole, through to the smoking population and then on to non-smokers, and now the major priority is to discourage women from smoking and young people being recruited to the smoking habit.

Some of these campaigns have been part of more integrated programmes aimed at the prevention of coronary heart disease. For example, the recent joint initiative 'Look after your heart' from the Department of Health and Social Security and the HEC (1986) which began in April 1987 has one of its immediate objectives to increase public awareness and support for healthy lifestyles as a goal for all with particular emphasis on contributing towards a decline in smoking. The campaign is aimed at everyone although it has a particular focus on working-class groups. This initiative is part of the HEC's Heartbeat 2000 programme where one of the overall aims is to meet the WHO strategy targets of reducing disease of the circulatory system in people under 65 by at least 15 per cent. The objective of this programme with regard to smoking is, together with the HEC's smoking education programme, to increase public awareness of evidence linking cigarette smoking and CHD and to promote non-smoking.

The second indirect policy strategy which the government has had some, if only a minimum involvement with, is controlling smoking in public places. The government has put some pressure on hospitals and health authorities to control smoking on health service premises as well as on British Rail and London Transport. The British government on the whole has been rather indifferent to this issue and perhaps any changes that have occurred have done so because of the concerns of the public (Wilkinson, 1986).

Summary of past and current policy in relation to smoking control

The piecemeal approach of the UK government towards smoking control has focused primarily on changing patterns of consumption through health education and, more recently, taxation. Little emphasis has been placed on direct intervention in the production process where voluntary agreements have been negotiated with the tobacco industry to regulate tobacco promotions and to develop a safer cigarette policy. Policies to control smoking in public places have been minimal.

Why has government policy taken this shape?

This section examines the policy process and attempts to explain why government policy has developed in the way that it has in this country.

As long ago as 1955 the government was made aware of the link between smoking and lung cancer (P. Wright, *The Times*, 7 January 1985). However, as was shown in the previous section, no real momentum in the development of a policy occurred until the 1970s. Government's relative inaction in the light of the availability of evidence linking smoking and ill-health was because of what Taylor (1984) has referred to as the smoke ring. The smoke ring is the ring of political and economic interests which has protected the tobacco industry and these interests include the government, the media and the addicted smoker. Taylor (1984) has given a detailed account of how these interests have influenced or perhaps restricted smoking control policy in this country; however, the major forces will be outlined briefly here. There are two and these are:

(i) the political strength of vested interests in tobacco manufacture and promotion in this country, e.g. tobacco companies and other interests vested in cigarette promotion such as newspapers and cinemas;
(ii) the confusion of interests within the government because:
    (a) the dependence on revenue from taxation of tobacco;
    (b) other government departments have interests in the maintenance of tobacco such as the Department of Employment.

Quite simply, those individuals or groups within or outside

government intent on developing a more 'interventionist' policy for government, such as direct controls over tobacco promotion, have had to struggle with powerful interests within and outside government. This is one of the reasons why government policy in this area has tended to try to influence the pattern of consumption mainly through trying to persuade smokers to change their behaviour.

Given these strong vested interests it is surprising that the government has taken any part in the development of policy towards smoking controls. The major reason why it has taken some action is due to the pressure of the anti-smoking lobby. The activities of individuals as well as the government-funded pressure group ASH may have been important, although one of the major influences, particularly in ensuring the 'problem of smoking' reached and stayed on the policy agenda was the publication of a series of reports on smoking and health by the Royal College of Physicians (1962, 1971, 1977, 1983a). The impact of these reports is difficult to assess, although some action directly followed the publication of the first two. In both cases it appeared to lead to the industry anticipating government action and thus agreeing to voluntarily adopt self-regulating measures. Each of the reports received wide publicity throughout the media and in each the government was exhorted to take sterner and more direct action.

The medical profession have recently taken a higher profile although this time through the BMA. In 1984, the BMA started its anti-smoking campaign which was directed at stopping tobacco advertising and the promotion of cigarettes through sponsorship (Wilkinson, 1986).

The effectiveness of government policy

To assess the effectiveness of government policy one must define what the aim of the policy is although the piecemeal nature of the policy suggests that defining objectives in this instance is difficult. Ideally, a comprehensive policy involving the government might aim to provide an environment where there was no pressure to smoke and smoking was not the norm. However, whatever the approach, one of the major indications of success would be a reduction in consumption.

Bearing in mind the difficulties in enforcing and regulating the legislative measures and the voluntary agreements the figures on changes in consumption over the last 15 years suggest that this piecemeal package of measures has had some success. In 1972, 52 per cent of the male and 41 per cent of the female population in Great Britain were smokers. However, by 1986 the proportion of adult male smokers fell by almost one-third to 35 per cent and that of women by about one-fifth to 31 per cent. The reasons for this decrease are twofold. Fewer people are starting to smoke and more people are giving up.

The profile of the current smoker is someone who is more likely to be male, to be aged between 20 and 60 and to come from social classes IV (semi-skilled occupations) and V unskilled-occupations. The social class differences remain marked, even though there has been a reduction in all the classes. The gender difference has been much reduced and there is only a marked gender difference in the 60+ age group and this is because most of the women in this age group never started to smoke. The age differences are small apart from 16–19 years and 60+ where there is a lower prevalence of smoking than in the other age groups. Between 1972 and 1984 all age groups showed a substantial fall although between 1982 and 1984 smoking prevalence among women rose in the age group 16–19. So for the first time more women aged 16–19 in 1984 smoked (32 per cent) than did men of the same age (19 per cent). No other age group showed an increase in prevalence.

There has, however, been a less dramatic reduction in the average consumption per smoker. For example, for male smokers the average weekly cigarette consumption was 120 in 1972, rose to 124 in 1976 and in 1984 fell to 115. However, for women the average weekly cigarette consumption in 1980 was 87, rose to 102 in 1982, and in 1984 declined slightly to 96.

This reduction in cigarette consumption over the last decade has been claimed to represent one of the few success stories in health promotion. However, as there has been little evaluative work it is difficult to judge whether it is due to this package or one measure within the package or due to a range of other factors. Some of the health education campaigns carried out in the mass media in the 1970s were evaluated and the results showed that the campaigns had little effect on smoking behaviour, at least in the short term (Calnan, 1982). The apparent failure of these mass-media campaigns could be put down to the lack of a large investment by the government, at least compared to the investment in pro-cigarette advertising by the tobacco industry. However, it might be expecting too much of these mass-media campaigns in that their major purpose may be only to set the 'agenda' and to help create a climate where smoking is socially unacceptable.

Townsend (1987) has argued that the price increases in cigarettes due to the substantial increases in tax between 1980 and 1984 were responsible for about half of the 20 per cent reduction in cigarette smoking during that period. The other half of the reduction was, according to Townsend, due to health education. However, these claims, particularly the one about the impact of health education, appear to be speculative. The recent health education programmes have been aimed at the younger age groups and there is little evidence of a more marked fall in this age group. Nor do the changes in cigarette consumption appear to be due to other smoking control strategies operating at the regional, district or professional levels as there is little evidence of a comprehensive policy.

The drop in consumption may have been due to a range of other factors such as the publicity given to the series of reports on smoking and health prepared by the Royal College of Physicians. Also, it might be due to broader changes such as the increasing interest in health amongst the population as a whole which reflects the trend towards individualism, self-reliance and individual responsibility.

There is also evidence which suggests that the government safer cigarette policy has been successful in that there has been a drop in the standard tar content of cigarettes and there has been a shift from high to low tar cigarettes (Calnan, 1984). However, from the point of view of reduction in CHD this policy is of little benefit and it would be of more value if this policy included reduction in other harmful constituents such as carbon monoxide.

In summary, the UK government has tended to opt for persuasion and self-regulation in its approach to the control of smoking rather than direct intervention. Only very recently has it favoured fiscal policy as a public health measure. The effectiveness of these policies adopted by the UK government is difficult to assess, although there has been a significant reduction over the last ten years in the proportion of smokers in the population. However, there are still marked social class differences in prevalence and smoking levels amongst the younger age groups are still high and, amongst younger women, are beginning to increase.

What could the government do?

The previous sections have suggested that even if the British government wished to, there may be a number of difficult economic and political obstacles to overcome if a comprehensive smoking control policy was to be developed by the government. However, if these obstacles are to be overcome, what policies should the government adopt?

Various policy options have been suggested although there is some consensus amongst agencies about which are most important. *The Canterbury Report* (Health Education Council, 1984) in its recommendations suggested a need to adopt taxation policies which kept the price of cigarettes above inflation as well as the introduction of legislation to ban cigarette promotion and advertising. The latter policy is particularly aimed at controlling the recruitment of young people to the smoking habit. Both these recommendations were supported by a recent report of a WHO expert committee (WHO, 1984), although this committee also advocated restrictions on smoking in public places and on public transport and the encouragement of diversification in the tobacco industry so that the industry can cope with a decline in tobacco production. Both reports recommended that product modification (safer cigarettes) should not be advocated as far as CHD is concerned.

Given that these policies have been recommended, what is the evidence to show that they are effective?

Fiscal policy

A government can attempt to control tobacco consumption through controlling subsidies for tobacco (Roemer, 1982). Alternatively, it can raise prices through taxation. The latter appears to be a more popular measure and the government can do this in three main ways:

(i) an overall progressive increase in taxation with the clear, health-related objective of reducing consumption;
(ii) a differential system of taxation which favours cigarettes which are low in tar, nicotine and carbon monoxide;
(iii) the inclusion in the tax structure of a levy to finance a smoking education programme.

The balance of evidence from studies examining the relationship between consumption and price (Russell, 1973; Peto, 1974; Atkinson and Skegg, 1974; Maynard, 1986) suggests the existence of an inverse relationship although the degree of change both in the short and longer terms caused by different increases in the price of cigarettes is difficult to predict and so is the impact of price changes on 'heavy' and 'light' consumers of cigarettes. It appears that the influence of price rises is temporary and therefore there is a need for consistent increases in the price of cigarettes to maintain a consistent decline in consumption. The problem is estimating how large price increases should be. The price elasticity of demand for tobacco appears generally to be in the

0.2 to 0.5 range (Maynard, 1986). Thus, a 1 per cent increase in price reduces consumption by 0.2 to 0.5 per cent. Maynard (1986) suggests that short-term price elasticity is probably higher, although he also suggests that there is the danger with large price increases of smokers merely switching to consumption of cheaper drugs such as alcohol.

One of the other problems with attempting to reduce cigarette consumption through large increases in prices is that poorer groups may be hardest hit. This is further compounded by the marked social class differences in the prevalence of smoking. The dependent nature of cigarette smoking, be it pharmacological, psychological or cultural, might mean that a smoker would give up other goods to continue smoking at the same level. Little is known about social class-specific price elasticities although Townsend (1987) suggests that price elasticity specific to low income groups is high and thus the decrease in real price of cigarettes prior to 1980 effectively increased the smoking levels of lower socio-economic groups relative to social classes I (professional occupations) and II (semi-professional occupations). Evidence on age-specific elasticity is also difficult to find although Maynard (1986) suggests that price elasticity amongst younger age groups may be higher than average and thus high price increases may be an effective instrument for reducing the take-up of smoking in this age group.

Also, as Godfrey and Maynard show (1988), the impact of a consistent increase in tobacco prices while reducing consumption can also reduce employment. Thus, a 10 per cent increase in tax each year could be estimated to result in a fall of 3,700 jobs in the tobacco industry. However, as the actions point out, job creation resulting from a shift in consumption patterns will offset these effects on employment.

Large increases in the price of cigarettes are said to have significant economic costs. One of these is in the loss of government revenue obtained by the taxation of cigarettes although the value of tobacco revenues has generally fallen. However, it has been shown (Atkinson and Townsend, 1977) that the low price elasticity of the demand for cigarettes means that large increases in price produce a gain rather than a loss in revenue. For example, Atkinson and Townsend (1977) claim that a 56 per cent increase in price would increase government revenue by 17 per cent as well as reducing smoking by 20 per cent. They also claim that a 40 per cent reduction in cigarette smoking produces a net increase in government revenue in that the savings from the reduction in expenditure on hospital inpatient stay, general practitioner consultations, sickness benefits and widows' benefits are larger than the costs incurred due to increases in expenditure on retirement pensions and health education. However, this has been contested by Leu and Schaub (1983) who challenge the claim that smoking imposes a large cost burden on health service systems. The results imply that life-time expenditure is higher for non-smokers than for smokers because smokers' higher annual utilisation rates are over-compensated for by non-smokers' higher life expectancy.

Ten years later, Townsend (1987), in an assessment of her predictions, suggests that during that period the real price was raised by 18 per cent, about a third of what was asked for; there was a limited investment in health education and little was done to restrict advertising. However, Townsend (1987) argues the result of this dual policy was to reduce consumption by nearly 20 per cent with 12 per cent due to health education and 8 per cent to the price increases. Townsend predicts that a further 20 per cent rise in price together with continued health education and restrictions on advertising would result in a further 20 per cent reduction in smoking, without loss of revenue.

Others have tended to suggest the economic benefits of a reduction in smoking amongst the population are not as great as some claim. For example, Cohen (1984) attempted to estimate the economic consequences of the emergence of a non-smoking generation. He estimated that there would be 70,000 fewer premature deaths due to smoking and, using a crude economic analysis, he showed that a reduction in smoking would save the government £1,400 million in terms of costs of sickness absence and health care but the government would lose £3,000 million in tobacco revenue. While over 26,000 jobs would be lost in the tobacco industry, Cohen suggests that these job losses would be minimised by the diversification activities of the tobacco companies. In conclusion, while Cohen argues that in terms of economic indicators considered, the pro-smoking lobby has the strongest argument, he states that a final judgement on whether smoking is a good or bad thing cannot solely be made on the basis of such a quantitative investigation, but will have to accommodate such 'intangibles' as the pleasure derived by smokers and the annoyance caused to non-smokers.

Controls over tobacco advertising

Controls over tobacco advertising in the UK have, as has already been shown, been implemented through voluntary agreements between the tobacco industry and the government. However, evidence has suggested that voluntary controls have less impact on tobacco consumption than legislative controls. For example, Cox and Smith (1984), using an econometric model of demand for tobacco, analysed the impact of legislative and voluntary controls on smoking trends in a group of 15 countries between 1962 and 1980. The results indicated that, after allowing for price and income effects, those countries which have adopted legislative controls over smoking have reduced and disrupted national tobacco consumption more than those countries where only voluntary controls are in evidence.

The specific legislative control that is of interest here is control over tobacco advertising and of prime importance here is whether such a ban is effective or not. Studies examining this issue have taken two forms. First, there are those econometric studies which have examined the relationship between cigarette advertising and the demand for cigarettes. No hard conclusions emerge from these studies given that some report that advertising has had a significant effect on the expansion of tobacco sales (McGuiness and Cowling, 1975), and others argue that there is little relationship between advertising and demand for tobacco (Fujii, 1980). However, as Cox argues (1984), it is quite mistaken to conclude from this that advertising may have only small effects; the existence of advertising on any large scale may help support a climate which portrays smoking as socially acceptable.

The second type of study involves a direct evaluation of the impact of legislation controlling advertising. For example, Bjartvert (1977) analysed smoking habits during the first year after implementation of the Norwegian Tobacco Act, 1975. The passing of this Act included a total ban on all advertising of tobacco products; legislation to label all packets with symbols and text pointing out dangers; and prohibitions of sale or handover to persons under the age of 16 years. The results showed that in Norway the adult per capita consumption fell by 2.7 per cent in 1975–76. This change was most marked in males, with a drop from 52 per cent to 48 per cent of smokers within a period of six months. No change in per capita consumption was found for women. In Oslo, there was a fall in smoking amongst men from 60 per cent to 45 per cent and daily consumption fell from 16.7 units to 14.4 units. The drop was most marked amongst the female population who were aged 15 to 21 years. These results suggest that the legislation is having an impact even at this early stage. More recent evidence supports this conclusion in that the smoking rate in 14-year-old boys dropped from 16 per cent (1973) to 13 per cent (1980) and from 17 per cent to 11 per cent for 14-year-old girls (Robson *et al.*, 1982). This trend has also been reported in the age group 16–20 years ten years after the legislation was created (Bjartvert, 1986).

Evidence from France where, in 1976, tobacco advertising was banned in the media, in places of entertainment and other public places, on posters and bill-boards and other signs, also suggests there has been a reduction in consumption (Roemer, 1982). In Finland, where there has been a ban on all forms of tobacco advertising, the smoking rate in 14-year-olds dropped from 19 per cent (1973) to 8 per cent (1979) (Robson *et al.*, 1982) although since then the trend has levelled-off (Lempo and Vertio, 1986).

The balance of evidence suggests that a ban on tobacco advertising can, probably in combination with a range of other measures, lead to a modest fall in cigarette consumption, particularly among the younger age groups. Certainly, the downward trends in smoking habits in Norway can only be attributed to a package of measures including price rises as it is impossible to single out individual measures and draw conclusions as to their effects in isolation.

There is some evidence to suggest it might not be necessary to ban tobacco advertising. Godfrey (1986) reports studies in the USA which have shown that a policy of having the same number of health messages as tobacco advertisements or having more prominent health messages within an advertisement may be more effective in reducing consumption than putting a limit to advertising expenditure.

Controls over smoking in public places

Control over smoking in public places has become of increasing importance as a measure which governments might adopt, mainly because of the attention given to the increasingly strong evidence of a link between passive smoking and lung cancer rather than CHD. Certainly, it is a measure that might be favoured by those who place great emphasis on the freedom of the individual and who are antagonistic towards more direct government intervention through fiscal policy or controls on tobacco promotion. It is a measure which relies heavily on the support of the general public which, according to some commentators (Wilkinson, 1986) would encourage it in Great Britain at present.

Sweden and the United States have implemented policies for controls over smoking (Wilkinson, 1986) in public places although such a measure is difficult to evaluate. Evidence could be collected on the consequences for passive smoking and also whether the controls reduce smoker's consumption.

Summary and conclusions

The evidence has suggested that a package of measures including large increases in the price of cigarettes, health education campaigns and legislative control over tobacco advertising could be very effective methods of reducing cigarette consumption. Certainly the analysis has suggested it would be more effective than the piecemeal approach offered by the British government so far.

Recent government intervention in Britain has favoured fiscal policy rather than control of tobacco manufacture or promotion, mainly because it is easier for the government to pursue simple bureaucratic procedures for regulating tobacco consumption than entering into a more complex relationship to control production. The brief analysis of various aspects of the policy-making procedures suggests that even if governments wanted increased direct control over the tobacco industry they would have to overcome the powerful interests within and outside the government (Milio, 1985). The difficulty of overcoming these obstacles should not be underestimated as a recent analysis of the development of smoking control policy in Finland (Lempo and Vertio, 1986) has shown. For example, in their discussion about the major issues in political decision-making which surrounded the introduction of legislation they state:

> Even in Finland, which is a small country with marginal significance to the world market, the tobacco industry fought with all its force at all stages of the battle to water down all proposals which were seen to be effective . . . the hardest political issues were (i) the ban on advertisements and sales promotion; (ii) the setting of upper limits for harmful substances in the yields of tobacco products, and the classification of them as 'very harmful' or 'harmful'; (iii) any proposals for effective price policies.

The struggle with vested interests was not just confined to the political process involved with getting the legislation onto the Statute books but also extended to the implementation of the policy. For example, the attempts to increase real prices to support other measures were contested by the Treasury on the grounds that it would run counter to the government's anti-inflationary policy. This led authors (Lempo and Vertio, 1986) to conclude:

> Those working with smoking policy in Finland generally find price policy an area where no progress has been made over the years, an area where short-term and narrowly-conceived economic policies overrun longer-term health interests.

Clearly, then, in the development of a coherent smoking control policy which is a central role for the government, policy-makers have come to terms with the realities of the economics of tobacco. The tobacco economy, while being a growing sector in developing countries, is a declining industry in affluent countries such as Britain. Milio (1985) puts forward a broad strategy for coping with these economic changes in tobacco which also attempts to incorporate a health promotion policy. This strategy has two general strands. The first is educational and will involve presenting to policy-makers and the media the smoking/health issue in the light of changing economic conditions. The second involves changes in the environment to improve the feasibility of policy measures for planning changes or transitions in the tobacco economy.

CONTROL OVER FOOD CONSUMPTION AND DIET

This second section focuses on government policy in relation to the control of dietary factors associated with an increased risk of CHD. The government has the option of allocating funds to the National Health Service for screening for blood pressure and serum cholesterol. Alternatively, the government could focus on primary prevention by trying, on a population basis, to reduce the determinants of elevated blood pressure and serum cholesterol. The evidence suggested that fat consumption (mainly saturated) was a major determinant of serum cholesterol levels and obesity, salt and alcohol consumption were significant influences on blood pressure levels. Thus, this analysis will focus on the control of these dietary factors leaving aside alcohol which will be considered in a later section.

UK government policy: past and present

The previous analysis of smoking policy showed that it was the link between smoking and lung cancer that brought the issue of smoking and health to the government's attention with concern about coronary heart disease following on afterwards. The UK government's interest in food policy, nutrition and health dates back to the 1920s. However, it was CHD and its links with diet through fat consumption that was the major reason why of late the government has shown increasing interest in diet and its consequences for health. The link between diseases and other dietary elements such as fibre and sugar has only very recently reached the policy agenda.

The Ministry of Agriculture, Food and Fisheries has the government's responsibility to control the quality of food available to the public, particularly composition and labelling. The Department of Health focuses mainly on the health-related aspects of food policy. It is through the DHSS Committee on the Medical Aspects of Food Policy (COMA) that much of government policy about diet and CHD has been reported. Certainly, MAFF are involved in the debate about food and health in that they are represented on COMA; however, concerns about health appear to compete with a range of other interests to get on to their policy agenda.

During the 1970s there was a series of government policy documents on diet and health and a number specifically on diet and CHD. For example, the 1974 COMA Committee on Heart Disease and Stroke recommended less consumption of fats, saturated fats, cholesterol and calories. No mention was made of alcohol and polyunsaturated fats. This report was followed by a number on prevention although the next one to focus on diet and its implications for CHD was the discussion booklet *Eating for Health* (DHSS, 1978). Amongst the recommendations was the need to cut down on sweet foods and fatty meat, butter, saturated fats, sugars, salt and alcohol as well as to reduce smoking. On the other hand, the booklet recommended eating more wholegrain bread, potatoes, vegetables, fruit and fibres and more exercise. However, when laying out their dietary recommendations, emphasis is placed on the individual's responsibility for maintaining a balanced diet. No mention is made of policies on food production and processing or establishing dietary goals to which food or the agricultural industries could adhere.

A similar pattern of recommendations was found in the DHSS report on heart disease published in 1984. However, three years later there was a substantial change in approach in the proposals put forward by the DHSS report of the COMA Committee (DHSS, 1984). Before these proposals are discussed in detail it is important to identify why there had been a change in approach at this time. There are at least two important factors. First, within the international scientific community there had been considerable debate and emerging consensus not only that dietary factors were causally associated with CHD, but that there should be generally a switch away from saturated to polyunsaturated fats. For example, in the United States the struggle against the epidemic of CHD had begun in the 1960s and by 1977 a set of specific targets or dietary goals was laid down. The McGovern goals suggested that 30 per cent of calorific intake should be from fats with 10 per cent from polyunsaturated fats. This report was followed by the WHO (1982) report on the prevention of CHD which recommended the need for governments to develop dietary goals and to adopt a population approach.

The second element which shaped the COMA proposals was the report of the National Advisory Committee on Nutrition Education in 1983. The NACNE Committee had been set up in 1979. The brief of the NACNE Committee was to identify deficiencies in the British diet and suggest remedies for them. The findings and recommendations of NACNE were seen in this country to be quite radical but compared with other countries were quite moderate. Its main conclusions were that the British food supply contained an excess of total fats, saturated fats, added sugars and salt and lacked fibre. It recommended specific long-term targets which included a cut in total fats by a quarter (30 per cent of total calories) and a halving of saturated fats (10 per cent of total calories). The Committee also rejected the previous approach of exhortation to individuals to eat in moderation by setting out specific targets within a plan for a healthy food supply which would need the government, the scientific community and industry each playing a full role.

The NACNE Committee's findings and recommendations, in spite of attempts to delay and stop them (Walker and Cannon, 1984), set the agenda for the COMA report as they were widely read and generally accepted. However, it was claimed that the NACNE report was disowned by the government and great emphasis was placed instead on the COMA proposals (Walker and Cannon, 1984).

Before the recommendations of the report are discussed it is necessary to outline the perspective adopted by the report which is well-illustrated by the following extract:

> Diet is a matter to be decided by individuals and by families after consideration of its possible bearing on health and of such guidance as may be available. So far as we are aware no government has attempted to enforce recommendations relating to nutrition and cardiovascular diseases by direct legislation. It seems likely that

> legislation based on agricultural policy and on economic policies connected with the production of food and with the sale of food and drink, may have a significant indirect effect on nutrition in relation to cardiovascular disease.
>
> If diet is to be decided by individuals then it is necessary that some foods and drinks should carry sufficient information about their composition to enable members of the public who wish to adjust their intake of particular dietary components to do so. Where such adjustments will be facilitated by making available alternative forms of certain goods, agricultural policy should not discontinue their availability.

The recommendations of the Committee were directed at the public, at medical practitioners, at health educationalists, at producers, manufacturers and distributors of food and drink and caterers and at the government. The recommendations to the public emphasised greater consumption of wholegrain cereal, wholegrain bread, vegetables, fruit, lean meat and poultry, fibres and starch and the adoption of regular exercise. On the other hand, they recommended less consumption of cakes, biscuits, fatty meats/meat produce, full fat milk, butter, salt, cigarettes and recommended that fats should not exceed 35 per cent of calorie intake and saturated fats should not exceed 15 per cent. No specific recommendations for change in the consumption of polyunsaturated and monounsaturated fatty acids were made although they recommended that the P:S ratio might be increased to approximately 0.45.

The more interesting recommendations, at least from a policy point of view, were those aimed at the government and the industry. The industry was invited to provide the consumer with more information by specifically printing information on containers or wrappers about fat content and percentage by weight of saturated, polyunsaturated and fatty acids; it was also recommended that there be a greater availability to the general public of low fat/low salt products. The recommendations to government suggested that:

> Consultations should take place between the relevant government departments and the producers, manufacturers and distributors of food and drink and caterers which will lead to legislation and to codes of practice to improve public knowledge of the composition of foods, improve public awareness of the alcohol content of alcoholic drinks and lead to the provision of alternative preparation of some food with lower contents of saturated and of trans fatty acid and/or common salt.

The report also recommended that consideration should be given to ways and means of encouraging the production of leaner carcasses in sheep, cattle and pigs as well as thinking of ways and means of removing from the common agricultural policy those elements of it which may discourage individuals and families from implementing recommendations for dietary change.

The response of the government to this report was the recommendation that the Joint Advisory Committee on Nutrition Education turn the scientific evidence in the report into practical guidelines on a sensible, healthy diet for families throughout the UK. This they did (HEC, 1985) in a short booklet entitled 'Eating for a healthier heart' which gave information about fat and suggested how families could change meals to decrease fat consumption.

The government thus responded to the recommendations for health education to the public and the recommendations for leaner carcasses, have been taken forward. Also the food labelling issue has been taken up and guidelines were published by MAFF in 1987/8. These proposals require food to be labelled with fat contents only although manufacturers can go further if they so wish. The form recommended by MAFF, for energy, fat, protein and carbohydrate, does not allow people to distinguish between the complex carbohydrate which they have been encouraged to eat and simple sugars of which they have been advised not to increase consumption.

Further health education about diet to the public has been made available in the recent DHSS/HEC (1986) campaign 'Look after your heart' where emphasis has been on increasing public awareness and support for the adoption of healthier eating and the need to avoid obesity. It is not evident what information on diet will be the basis for this dietary change although the emphasis is on changing behaviour through persuasion and education. However, MAFF and DHSS recently carried out a dietary and nutritional survey of adults aged 16 to 64 in Great Britain. The survey will provide information about patterns of food consumption nationwide.

The government has also been involved in another CHD prevention programme involving attempts at dietary change through its funding of the Health Education Council. However, the role of the Health Education Council will be discussed at the end of this chapter.

Summary of past and current policy in relation to food and diet

CHD has been the major focus for government policy on food and health in this country although the formulation of policy documents has only spanned just over a decade. Government policy about smoking control was described as piecemeal and non-directive. Similar conclusions can be made about its involvement in dietary control. It is only very recently that the policy documents have agreed on a coherent policy involving not just the consumer but also the government and industry. The implementation of these proposals has been limited and has tended to be restricted to education of the consumer. However, there have been some recent attempts by government to reduce the fat content of food through influencing the food supply. For example, a new government regulation which came into effect in January 1986 has stopped the subsidy for the production of very fat lambs, although it continues to treat lean and moderately fat lambs alike. A similar regulation has been introduced to curtail production of very fat beef, although when combined with Common Agricultural Policy (CAP) mechanisms of intervention buying it can leave the consumer without access to leaner cuts of meat which have been bought by the government.

Why has government policy taken this shape?

There is a dearth of documentary evidence about the factors that shape the government's policy or non-policy on food and health. However, it is possible to build up albeit a superficial picture of why this particular approach has developed. The analysis of smoking policy showed how vested interests in tobacco production, along with the confusion of interests in the government, restricted government intervention although the power of the medical profession forced the problem onto the agenda. The relative inaction of government in this area compared with smoking may reflect the power of the interest groups which control the food supply in this country, particularly food manufacturers and producers. There is also considerable confusion of interests within the government, particularly between MAFF and DH, and also between the policies of the EEC, particularly CAP and the British government. In addition, there are the MPs who have constituency interests in the maintenance of the present food supply.

Certainly, there has been a series of reports by the medical profession, particularly by the Royal College of Physicians, although they have lacked the authority and commitment of the reports on smoking. This may be due to a lack of scientific evidence, and a belief that food was unimportant in the cause of disease. It was not until 1983 (Walker and Cannon, 1984) 'that the Lancet started a series of articles on nutrition, the changing scene which helped place nutrition on the medical profession's agenda.' The power of the interests groups and the confusion of interests within government is well reflected in the report of the findings of the NACNE Committee. For example, as Walker and Cannon (1984) state:

> The conflicting advice offered with NACNE at its first meeting was not because doctors and scientists on the Committee were in basic medical or scientific disagreement. Rather, the causes of disagreement and conflict were of a political, industrial and commercial nature. For example, there is a massive surplus of dairy products in Europe, and British meat and dairy-farmers are important people in Britain. In such circumstances, it is understandable that some members of NACNE whose jobs involve protecting the interests of farmers and of the food industry did not readily accept that British public should eat – and drink – a lot less fat. Fat, sugar and salt are profitable commodities – fresh cereals, vegetables and fruit less so.

There was also evidence (Walker and Cannon, 1984) that the publication of the NACNE report was delayed as a result of pressure placed on the DHSS by government representations and the food manufacturing industry.

The effectiveness of government policy

The almost complete lack of government policy, at least up until very recently, suggests that there is little benefit in examining data to assess their possible value. However, examination of changes is necessary in that it can show what has been achieved and what could be achieved in the future. There is little evidence available to assess the link between changes in diet and serum cholesterol or to changes in morbidity or mortality from CHD. However, there is evidence on changes in diet between the early 1960s up until the present time (CSO, 1989).

Table 2.1 shows that since 1961 consumption of milk, cream, butter and lard (which comes under All other fats) dropped dramatically. Between 1972 and 1980 (Walker, 1984), the P:S ratio had increased from 0.20 to 0.24 and this was mainly due to a fall in saturated fat intake rather than an increase in polyunsaturated fatty acids. Milk and butter are the major contributors to saturated fat intake but with regard to total

Table 2.1 Purchases[1] of selected foods for home consumption

Great Britain	*Indices of average quantities per person[2] per week, 1980 = 100*										
	1961	*1971*	*1976*	*1980*	*1981*	*1982*	*1983*	*1984*	*1985*	*1986*	*1987*
Type of food											
Milk and cream	114	113	111	100	97	96	94	94	90	91	89
Cheese	79	93	97	100	100	98	103	99	101	107	105
Eggs	126	123	111	100	100	95	96	87	85	82	78
Beef and veal	112	98	94	100	86	87	81	77	80	81	83
Mutton and lamb	150	120	93	100	94	80	86	74	73	67	59
Pork	47	74	70	100	92	97	85	80	84	88	77
Poultry	36	73	90	100	109	102	104	108	102	107	119
All other meats and meat products	98	105	98	100	102	103	103	99	100	100	98
Fish and fish products	119	107	95	100	103	105	107	102	102	108	106
Butter	153	137	127	100	91	78	81	71	70	56	53
Margarine	86	82	80	100	107	113	107	107	98	107	104
All other fats	76	87	82	100	97	104	99	100	104	123	117
Fresh potatoes	138	120	86	100	102	100	97	97	100	95	92
Other fresh vegetables[3]	101	99	92	100	98	95	94	92	90	99	94
Other vegetables and vegetable products[3]	61	78	92	100	105	107	107	105	114	121	120
Fresh fruit	83	96	88	100	96	90	94	91	89	98	97
Other fruit and fruit products	88	92	88	100	109	113	125	122	118	144	148
Bread, standard white loaves	165	137	121	100	100	99	95	92	89	76	73
Bread, brown and wholemeal	58	55	65	100	100	97	106	118	132	165	151
Cakes, biscuits, etc.	128	123	105	100	100	103	99	97	95	99	99
Sugar	162	141	109	100	99	92	88	82	75	72	67
Tea	139	117	108	100	97	99	100	88	85	85	83
Instant coffee	30	81	94	100	96	94	98	100	100	102	96

1 includes also the household consumption of 'free' foods, e.g. garden and allotment produce etc.
2 irrespective of age
3 includes tomatoes

Source: Central Statistical Office (1989)

fat intake they are equal contributors with oils, lard and mayonnaise.

More recent evidence (MAFF, 1987) has shown that between 1980 and 1986 the intake of saturated fats in the British diet continues to decline so that the P:S ratio has risen from 0.24 in 1980 to 0.35 in 1986 and the proportion of energy derived from saturated fatty acids has declined from 18.8 per cent in 1980 to 17.7 per cent in 1986. However, fat continues to provide between 42–43 per cent of the energy value of the household diet which is way above the target of 35 per cent recommended in the COMA report. A more recent national study of British adults (Gregory *et al.*, 1990) found that in 1987 fat provided 40.4 per cent and 40.3 per cent of food energy for men and women respectively and the P:S ratio for men and women was 0.40 and 0.38 respectively.

The major problem with much of this evidence is that it appears only to give a partial picture, in that while inside the home people are eating less saturated fat and more polyunsaturated fat, outside the home there are indications that a reverse trend is occurring (Rayner, 1989). Between 1977 and 1987 the average number of meals eaten per week outside the home in cafes, fast food outlets, at work, etc., increased by 17 per cent. Eating out, as Rayner points out (1989), tends to go hand in hand with consumption of high-fat foods. It is noticeable that consumption of chips increased from 21 grammes per person in 1976 to 41 grammes per person per day in 1986.

Despite these figures about food eaten outside the home there is still evidence of a change in the P:S ratio. This appears mainly to have been brought about by a switch from butter to margarine. Rayner(1989) identifies five possible explanations for the switches:

(i) The impact of price
(ii) The effects of income
(iii) Technological change in the food industry
(iv) Effects of other trends in food consumption
(v) Advertising and health education

The fall in the consumption of bread, higher expenditure on margarine compared with butter, improvement in taste and keeping of margarine may have increased margarine consumption, relative to butter. However, probably the two most important effects have been the price differentiates between the two products with the EEC/CAP policies keeping the price of butter artificially high. The other effect is the change in the public's attitude to food and health.

Other changes have been occurring in the dairy industry and other sections of the farming industry. As we have seen, liquid milk consumption has also been dropping with more milk being used for the manufacture of skimmed-milk powder mainly for animal feed. EEC policy has attempted to restrict over-production and on 1 April 1984 milk quotas were introduced. If the proposed quotas are met then 53 × 103 tonnes/year less dairy fat will be produced in the UK.

However, despite this, until recently, the price paid to the producers for butter-fat has been more than the price for milk protein and thus there had been little initiative to produce low fat milk. This policy appears to be contrary to consumer wishes in that there has been a shift away from high-fat to low-fat milk and about a quarter of the milk now sold has a reduced fat content.

So some changes in the dairy industry are taking place but as Wheelock and Fallows (1985) point out it is an industry which will have problems if the COMA recommendations are met. They show that the dairy industry would have to reduce its production by 130 × 103 tonnes of fat less per year compared with a current production of some 700 × 103 tonnes/year. One of the problems appears to be that the dairy industry has fewer opportunities for diversifying into low-fat products without cutting overall production.

In contrast, in the livestock industry, to meet COMA's dietary targets a cut in total meat consumption is not necessary. COMA recommended an overall reduction in fat consumption of around 175 tonnes which would mean a reduction in total meat consumption of 99 × 103 tonnes a year. This might be achieved by changing the fat content of meat consumed or shifting from one type of meat or cut of meat to another. For example, there has been a trend towards leaner pork. This trend has been facilitated by an efficient method of grading the fat content of carcasses and live animals. The trend towards leaner pork has been achieved by breeding, changes in feeding methods, and changes in animal husbandry.

In contrast, there has been no marked change in the fat content of beef over the last decade. Certainly, there is little incentive in the pricing policy to favour the production of leaner animals. The carcass grading system for beef has the effect of favouring the production of fatter animals. In addition, under the current system of subsidy payments for beef, administered under the CAP, farmers are paid more for fatter animals. This system has been slightly modified and from 1 April 1986 very fat animals have no longer qualified for payment. A similar payment system exists for lamb production although from 1 June 1986 some of the fatter carcasses have been ineligible for premiums.

More opportunities for diversification therefore exist in the livestock industry and there is also the possibility of shifting from one type of meat (beef) to poultry as a method of reducing fat consumption. However, it is claimed that (Wheelock, 1986) such a shift may not be justified as if excess fat is trimmed from red meat, then there is little difference in fat levels between red meat and chicken. Also, there has been a tendency for the fat content of poultry to increase and there has also been a rapid expansion in processed poultry products containing added fat.

What could be done?

To develop an effective dietary policy for the prevention of CHD it is important to find out what the major determinants of food consumption are in this country. Patterns of food consumption are probably determined by consumer demand as well as supply. Sanderson and Winkler (1983) have described the phases of production, distribution and consumption as the 'food chain' and have shown how each of these elements is linked in a chain of relationships. One end of the food chain is the producer of primary foodstuffs which is linked with the treaters of raw foodstuffs such as abattoirs or creameries. These are linked to the manufacturers who transform the raw foodstuff into a consumer product. Intermediaries such as advertising facilitate the flow of goods and consumers either purchase it for private consumption or caterers transform it for consumption.

The government or other agency could intervene at any of these points in the chain although for an effective policy to be developed it is important to find out which part of the chain has the most powerful influence on food consumption.

Obviously, the structure and nature of the food supply have an important influence on patterns of food consumption. However, it is important not to neglect the factors that shape consumer preferences. For example, a pricing policy might assume that economic factors are powerful influences on consumer choice although evidence from anthropological research suggests that there is a range of other factors that also has an influence. Thus, more research should examine the factors that shape individual and family patterns of food purchase, preparation and the type of meals consumed.

Various sets of recommendations have been put forward which specify the government's role in dietary control for the prevention of CHD. Perhaps the most coherent have been put forward in *The Canterbury Report* (HEC, 1984) which based its recommendations on the WHO expert committee which reported in 1982. Thirteen recommendations were made but the most significant were:

(i) DHSS to formulate national food and health policy which quantified dietary goals and guidelines as a basis for policy implementation by MAFF;
(ii) MAFF should oppose anti-food health elements in CHD;
(iii) MAFF should consider the following ways of reducing the fat, sugar and salt content of the national food supply by (a) adjusting the carcass grading systems for sheep, cattle and pigs to encourage farmers by incentives to produce lean carcasses; (b) examining and altering food regulations to provide opportunities for manufacturers to improve food composition and make foods compatible with nutritional objectives; (c) subsidise agriculture for health diet such as cereals and shift away from milk, fat and sugar production;
(iv) codes of practice drawn up by MAFF and food industry which set a series of targets aiming at a steady reduction in the amounts of saturated fat, sugar and salt entering the UK diet via processed food;
(v) food labelling should be improved either by voluntary codes of practice or legislation;
(vi) codes of practice should be set up to control marketing and advertising.

An additional element was added to this list by the recent WHO expert committee (WHO, 1986) which suggested a need for community education on a healthy diet to be integrated in other efforts to promote a healthy lifestyle.

Some countries have developed and implemented national food and health policies and have adopted similar policies to those recommended in *The Canterbury Report* (HEC, 1984). For example, in 1975 the Norwegian government approved a national nutrition policy. The basic approach of the policy is a rejection of coercive measures and encouragement of consumers to voluntarily alter their dietary habits. Specific dietary goals were set and they were to be met (Milio, 1981) by (a) public and professional education and research; (b) regulating the quality of food products, the assortments on retail store shelves and meal provision in public institutions; (c) the joint setting of producer and consumer prices, providing incentives for the more health-promoting types of food; and (d) institutional integration.

There was some, but only partial, success in the implementation of these policies as well as in the achievement of the objectives. For example, full nutrient labelling became extensive and the margarine industry agreed to continue to improve the fat quality of its product. Also, consumer price subsidies were shifted to favour skimmed milk over full-fat milk, poultry over pork, and margarine over butter. However, pricing policies were one of the most difficult to implement and during the period 1977–80 beef became cheaper in relation to disposable income and its consumption increased markedly. There was also an increase in sugar consumption. More recent figures (Milio, 1989) show that between 1979–87 while fish and grain prices were well above the average dairy produce and sugar showed a higher rate and fresh produce was at a relatively low rate of increase.

While some of the economic objectives were met during the period 1976–80 such as an increase in production of food grains and vegetables, there was less success in the dietary and health objectives. There were increases in consumption of vegetables, fruit, cereals and skimmed milk, although there was little change in pork, fish or potato purchase. Beef and sugar consumption went up but milk, margarine and other fats decreased. There was a slight drop in cardiovascular disease death rate between 1970 and 1974 and a marked decline (50 per cent) in dental decay among children.

It will be interesting to see what impact the Norwegian policy has had in the longer term. In terms of understanding the conditions that enabled the setting up of this policy, Milio (1989) identified three important elements:

(i) economic conditions give policies impetus, i.e. growing uncertainty of essential food imports led to need for self-sufficiency;
(ii) nutrition-health problems could be re-interpreted to interest groups and policy-making in the light of the recognised economic and political reality;
(iii) eased by implementation of policy decisions through recognised channels between the government and other agencies.

Milio (1989) concludes:

> Most of the policy's nutritional increases can be attributed to the actions of the Nutrition Council, which even with little strategic capacity, pursued its mandate in ways that were often strategically effective.

Finally, one country which has experienced a dramatic decline in mortality rates from CHD is the USA. At least part of this decline may have been due to primary prevention and its influence on risk factors such as diet. For example (Epstein, 1984), between 1963 and

1980 milk and cream consumption decreased by 24 per cent, butter consumption by 33 per cent, animal fats and oils by 39 per cent, while the consumption of vegetable fats and oils rose by 58 per cent and fish by 23 per cent. Clearly, these are marked changes and it would be reasonable to assume that they influenced serum cholesterol levels which in turn influenced CHD mortality rates. However, this assumption has been contested. For example, Pickard (1986) argues that during the period 1965 to 1982 the percentage of saturated fat in the American food supply only fell by 4 per cent from 37 per cent to 33 per cent. The fall in the consumption of animal fat was partially replaced by the increased intake of vegetable fat. Saturated fat as a percentage of total calorific intake only fell from 15 per cent in 1965 to 14 per cent in 1982. Pickard (1986) also argues that the decline in animal fat consumption had begun as far back as the turn of the century. For example, she shows that in 1909–13 the percentage of animal fat in the American food supply was 83 per cent compared with 66 per cent in 1965; 57 per cent in 1976 and 57 per cent in 1982. The implication of this is that the decline in CHD rates should have occurred much earlier if the claim that animal fat consumption is causally related to CHD mortality is to be sustained.

Milio (1989) follows a similar line to Pickard but puts forward different explanations. She argues that general nutrient and food trends often mask policy – relevant questions about who is buying and using which foods and where they are eating. She illustrates by showing that within the long-term drop in dairy product consumption per capita, cheese increase has doubled in the last 20 years, mainly through away-from-home eating habits and processed food rather than home use where it is declining.

Milio accounts for these patterns of food consumption in terms of changing patterns of social and economic life. These social changes include a rapid increase in single-parent households and in dual-career couples and families. She states 'In contrast to one-career families, for example, single households spend almost twice as much of their food dollar (66 per cent) away from home, and career couples, compared to similar ones with children spend 50 per cent more away from home, less on dairy products, and more on "convenience", time-saving home meals.'

These changes in social and economic arrangements, according to Milio, have stronger effects on food variations than age and gender and lead to increased consumption of cheese, butter, saturated vegetable oils, sodium and sweeteners that are relatively more available in restaurants, fast foods, processed and 'convenience' products than at home. However, amongst elderly groups who are mainly women, the food patterns are closer to the dietary guidelines because they have more direct control in food buying and preparation. So, as Milio points out, the apparent changing trends in USA patterns of food consumption are misleading and disguise different patterns of food consumption amongst different groups.

Milio (1989) also suggests in her comparison between Norway (Public Health) and USA (market economy) that it is difficult to identify the impact of food health policies on food consumption patterns in the USA. She states:

> Food and nutrition policies have been found to be piecemeal, influenced by political and commercial interests, and consequently inconsistent, tending to neutralize or confound support for healthy nutritional patterns. Conclusions to date are that a market approach to nutrition and health [is] guided by the 'invisible human' rather than public policy guiding governmental, commercial and other organized actions – cannot promote the potential health gains of the 'New Nutrition' for all sections of the population.

Thus, according to Milio (1989), changes in patterns of dietary consumption were inspired by changes in patterns of social and economic life and economic factors such as prices and incomes rather than coherent food health policies. She shows that the market–demand framework uses information dissemination as the chief policy tool. She states:

> Much of the information that reaches the U.S. public by farm–food industry has been shown to be interpretations favouring commercial interests. Often, when nutritionally improved products have appeared over the last 30 years they have been a result of the fortuitous merging of public and corporate self-interests.

In conclusion, Britain has been slow to develop a coherent food health policy although the developments which have taken place have mainly focused on the prevention of CHD. It is too early to judge how effective these policies have been although the overall approach is piecemeal at least compared with the more coherent and comprehensive policies adopted in countries like Norway.

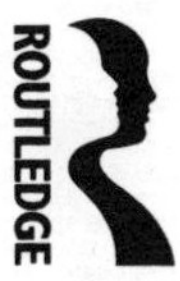

11 New Fetter Lane
London EC4P 4EE
Telephone: 071-583 9855
Fax: 071-583 4519

We have much pleasure in sending you the accompanying book for review

Title: Preventing Coronary Heart Disease

Author: Calnan

ISBN: Hb 0 415 04490 1
Pb

Publication Date: 1.8.91

Published Price: £ 35.00 Hb
£ Pb

A copy of the review would be greatly appreciated. Reviews should not appear in the press prior to the date of publication.
For further information please contact:

Chris Robertson

CONTROL OVER ALCOHOL CONSUMPTION

UK government policy: past and present

It must be emphasised that the focus here will be on those government policies aimed at controlling excessive alcohol use so as to influence physical health rather than those aimed at controlling the social and psychological effects of alcohol such as drinking and driving, drunkenness and public and domestic violence and the impact of heavy drinking on the individuals' lives and the lives of their families. To make such a distinction is in some ways artificial, particularly when the aim is to control excessive drinking whatever effect of drinking is the specific target of the policy. Even policies aimed at controlling drinking in specific situations, such as the legal control of drink when driving, may have spin-off effects on excessive drinking by reducing the range of circumstances in which drinking is legitimate. So the policies considered here will be those aimed at controlling excessive alcohol use with a specific focus on implications for physical ill-health. Certainly as was shown in the early part of the chapter, CHD has only recently been mentioned as one of the more harmful effects of alcohol and thus has not had a priority in policies for control.

It was argued in the previous section that, compared with the control of cigarette smoking, food and dietary policy has been, up until recently, relatively neglected. The same can be said of alcohol control policy. Alcohol problems did eventually arrive on the policy agenda in the 1960s (Baggott, 1986) but it was in response to the social problems of public drunkenness as well as the health problems associated with drink and driving and alcoholism. The response of the government to the problem was to expand the provision of service to cope with 'alcoholics'. However, by the late 1970s the emphasis in policy began to shift away from the provision of services to deal with 'problem drinkers' to an approach which aimed at the prevention of alcohol misuse through the control of the overall consumption of alcohol in society.

During the late 1970s three authoritative reports (Baggott, 1986) were published which emphasised the needs of government to counter the rise in alcohol consumption. The contents of these reports were in many respects ignored in the DHSS's consultative document (DHSS, 1981) entitled 'Drinking sensibly' which argued against the specific use of taxation and liquor licensing as instruments to regulate alcohol consumption.

There have, however, been some governmental interventions, although these interventions have not necessarily been inspired by public health motives. The availability of alcohol in terms of the number of permitted hours of drinking in licensed premises and legal age limits is more limited in the UK than in most other European countries. There is also legislation to limit drinking by motorists and there are voluntary restrictions of the marketing of alcoholic drinks. The advertising codes of practice operated by the Independent Broadcasting Authority and the Advertising Standards Authority regulate the advertising of alcohol. However, there have been no direct restrictions on the manufacture of alcoholic beverages and the real prices of alcoholic beverages are more heavily taxed in the UK than in most other European countries. The taxation system in the UK discriminates against spirits and in favour of beer. The philosophy behind this system seems to be primarily economic in that it is the most lucrative means of obtaining revenue without risking a drop in consumption.

The effectiveness of government policy

It is difficult to evaluate the impact of these measures particularly because of the problem of identifying whether the major influence on patterns of drinking is indigenous drinking practices or the controls over availability. The answer is that the two probably interrelate. By European standards, the per capita consumption of pure alcohol in the UK is low (Davies and Walsh, 1983) although the overall consumption of pure alcohol in the UK has increased over the last 20 years. Whilst beer remains the preferred beverage, the greatest increases have been in wine and spirit consumption (Calnan, 1982). Some recent evidence from the General Household Survey (OPCS, 1986b) suggests that this increase may be slowing down. Survey data about alcohol consumption are notoriously unreliable, particularly in terms of under-reporting. The GHS has, therefore, classified respondents into different types of drinker rather than attempting to measure actual alcohol consumption. The means of classification is the Quantity/frequency Index; respondents are asked how frequently they consume various kinds of alcoholic drink and how much of each they normally drink on any one occasion. Results show that the only consistent change has been a reduction in the proportion of men who are heavy drinkers from 25 per cent in 1978 to 20 per cent in 1984. However, there was also a small increase in the proportion of male and female frequent light drinkers. However, these data say little about overall consumption in the population and more recent data (CSO, 1989) show that between 1978 and 1987 the average number of units of alcohol consumed weekly increased for men but decreased for women (see Table 2.2).

Why has government policy taken this shape?

The government's policy towards the control over cigarette consumption was described as piecemeal. It would be fair to describe the government's approach to the control of alcohol use in the same way. Why, then, has the government refused to take direct action to control alcohol consumption? Baggott (1986) has identified four main political reasons for this government stance which are (i) the opposition of the

Table 2.2 Average number of units of alcohol consumed weekly, by age and sex, 1978 and 1987

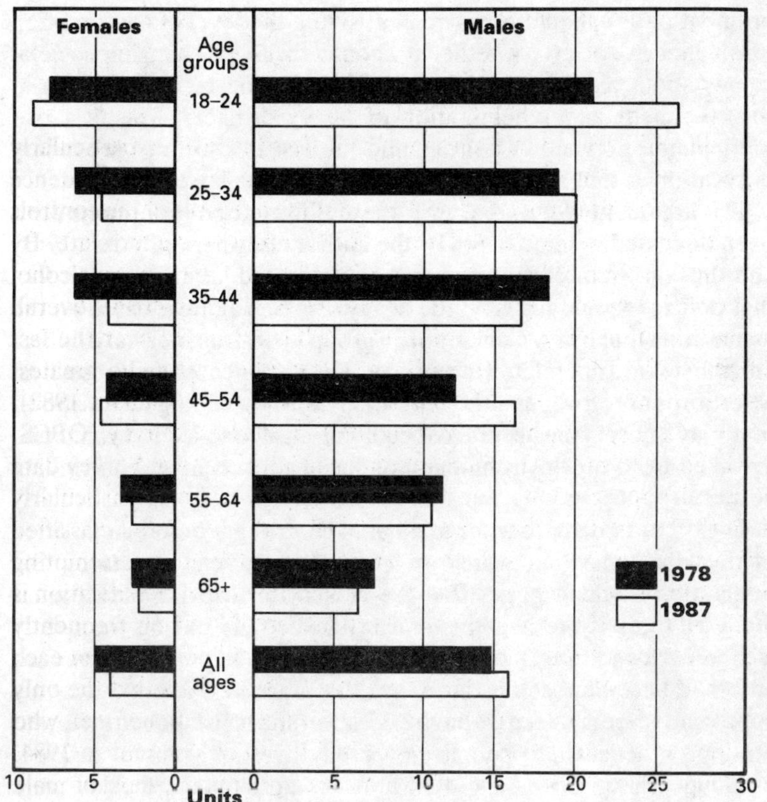

Source: Central Statistical Office (1989)

drinks industry whose power to influence government policy stems not just from its economic significance but also the support it receives from government departments such as MAFF; (ii) the opposition of government departments such as the Treasury who have responsibility for taxation policy and the Home Office who have responsibility for the licensing laws; (iii) the state of parliamentary, party and public opinion; and (iv) the weakness of the alcohol misuse lobby. Certainly, as was shown in the analysis of smoking control, powerful groups such as the medical profession are necessary if the powerful vested interests are to be countered.

What could the government do?

Before various control policies are considered, it is necessary to examine the theoretical evidence upon which various government policies could be based. The important question is whether government policy should focus on controlling the level of consumption of alcohol in society, whether it should focus on changing societal values about alcohol or whether it should allocate its resources to the treatment and rehabilitation of heavy drinkers. The first two are genuine prevention policies and the last is a form of secondary prevention in that it may reduce ill-health through treatment.

The arguments for and against these different policy options have been discussed in some depth by the author elsewhere (Calnan, 1982) and thus only a brief summary will be presented here. The argument that policies should focus on the heavy drinkers alone is based on the assumption that heavy drinkers are a group apart from normal drinkers and the two are not related in any way. The evidence to support such an assertion is not strong as although biological or psychological attributes may play a part in the process of becoming an alcoholic, they cannot be divorced from the environmental or social context in which drinking occurs.

The other two approaches to alcohol control are based on theories of drinking behaviour which are more sociological in nature. The integration model suggests that the reason for drinking problems in many cultures is the negative and mystical value put on the use of alcohol. Alcohol use is divorced from normal everyday life practices and thus becomes seen as an unhealthy practice. According to this approach, there is a need through education and legislation to integrate drinking practices into people's everyday lives and thus 'normalise' drinking. The policies suggested are, amongst others, the lowering of the legal drinking age, relaxing the licensing laws on availability of alcohol by increasing hours of drinking time, and educating young people in the use of alcohol in their everyday lives such as at mealtimes.

How effective the 'integration' approach is depends to a large extent on the indices of outcome used to evaluate it. For example, a study evaluating the impact of the licensing laws in Scotland (Duffy and Plant, 1986) shows no appreciable effect on alcohol-related morbidity or mortality, but an increase in the rate of convictions for drunkenness. Thus, the 'integration' approach may be valuable for controlling 'drunkenness' and the social problems associated with it, but do little to reduce ill-health. The latter argument is further supported (Davies and Walsh, 1983) by international comparisons. In countries where drink appears to be integrated with everyday life, such as France, Italy and Spain, compared with other Europeans countries where there are stronger controls on the availability of alcohol, the rates of heavy daily alcohol consumption and the rates for death from cirrhosis of the liver are relatively high.

The third approach suggests, in contrast to the integration theory, that the level of consumption of alcohol in a society is directly associated with the prevalence of heavy drinking. The implication of such an approach is that central government can influence heavy drinking by attempting to control overall consumption of alcohol. This approach, too, has its drawbacks although it is an approach which has received increasing support and it is the rationale on which many government alcohol control measures are based.

A range of alcohol control measures has been used in different countries and these have included age limitations, type and frequency of outlet and hours for sale, marketing and profit seeking, monopoly and licensing systems, education and price and taxation. Some of these measures, as has been pointed out, have been adopted in Britain but not necessarily for reasons of public health. The effectiveness of these measures has been reviewed elsewhere in some detail (Calnan, 1982). The outcome of this review suggests that evidence to support the idea that limitation of the hours of sale of alcohol as found in the UK is an effective alcohol control measure is difficult to find. Also, there was little evidence to show that monopoly systems were more effective than licensing systems. However, findings do suggest that age limits may well exercise a restraining influence and that lowering the legal drinking age may lead to an increase in consumption and alcohol problems if people begin to start drinking at a younger age. There is some evidence to show that a drop in consumption of alcohol in countries such as Sweden is due to controls over marketing and production, although the one genuine control measure appears to involve changes in price through taxation. However, changes in price through taxation appear to have different effects according to beverage type. Spirits have a greater price elasticity than beer and thus governments favour differential taxation of spirits because it does not lead to a loss in revenue but may also control 'drunkenness' from spirits drinking. In terms of public health measures such an approach may only be legitimate if spirit drinking creates greater long-term health problems than beer (Calnan, 1982).

EXERCISE AND OTHER RISK FACTORS

The major focus of policy in this area has been on control of smoking, diet and alcohol. However, other risk factors were identified in the first chapter, such as lack of exercise, stress and social and economic circumstances which up until now have been neglected. It is hardly surprising, given the current emphasis in government policy on individual responsibility, that social and economic influences on health status have been ignored. However, current policy does involve encouragement of individuals to adopt healthy lifestyles, thus there has been increasing emphasis on educating people to carry out regular exercise. It must be remembered that, unlike smoking, with food and alcohol there are no vested interests constraining the provision of exercise facilities, and government policy, or the lack of it, is a clear statement of the interest and priority placed on this issue.

The Department of the Environment has the government's responsibility for promoting exercise and sports facilities and it sponsors the Sports Council to encourage participation in sports and recreational activities to enhance health and fitness. However, the £37 million allocated in 1987 to the Sports Council has been cut recently, in real terms, by £3 million (National Forum of CHD Prevention, 1988). Also, the recent decision to privatise local authority leisure and sports facilities may not help the Sports Council's policy to encourage mass participation in sport.

It is difficult to gauge how much the provision of recreation and sports facilities has changed over the last decade. It has been claimed (Tracey, 1987) that the number of sports centres in the UK has increased from 24 in 1973 to over 1,000 in 1987. It has also been claimed that a parallel increase has occurred in relation to the provision of swimming pools, running tracks and other sporting facilities.

Despite this apparent improvement in provision of exercise facilities, figures from the General Household Surveys suggest that only 40.6 per cent of the population in 1983 reported that they participated once a month or more often in outdoor sport which included walking (2 miles or more) and rambling and 27.3 per cent were engaged in some kind of indoor sport. The latter included darts and snooker. However, even though this participation represents minimal involvement by a minority since 1977 there has been increased involvement, particularly in indoor sports.

There are also marked variations in participation by socio demographic groups. Participation declines steadily with age and male participants outnumber females by almost two to one. The gap between the sexes is particularly marked for outdoor sports but is narrowing for indoor sports due to the increase in keep fit and dance programmes.

Evidence from other sources (Collins, 1987) shows that there are continuing gaps between rich and poor in opportunities for playing sport and these gaps are not closing. As sport is income-related, retirement and unemployment generally lead to lower participation apart from the cheaper sports. Collins reports that the classic stereotypes basically continue in practice, with squash and golf as high income activities, swimming as a middle income activity and soccer, keep fit, bowls and fishing as lower income activities.

In summary, it was suggested earlier that regular, strenuous exercise could lead to a fall in CHD risk. The evidence presented here is that only a minority of the population appears to be carrying out such levels of exercise and that participation is lower amongst those groups (low income) at most risk.

SPECIFIC CHD PREVENTION POLICIES

The policies, or lack of them, described previously have focused on the control of risk factors which may or may not be specifically directed at coronary heart disease. However, there have been some government initiatives which have been specifically aimed at the prevention of cardiovascular disease. It is possible to identify at least three initiatives. First, it funds through the Department of Health (DH) the Coronary Prevention Group (CPG). The CPG has a number of different functions, one of which is to work as a pressure group lobbying in parliament or in other organisations with the objective of getting CHD prevention onto the political agenda and keeping it there.

Second, the government funds the Health Education Authority which has carried out a series of campaigns. *The Beating Heart Disease* pamphlet which was published in 1982 is the best illustration of the

HEC's programme which was directly aimed at CHD prevention. It is a pamphlet which is still currently available and has been widely distributed. It gives information about 'what heart disease is', 'how it is caused' and 'what can be done about it?' It exhorts individuals to reduce their risk of getting CHD by not smoking; eating less fat, salt and sugar, but eating more fibre; drinking less alcohol, carrying out more exercise and learning how to deal with stress. It gives some information about how this can be achieved. It also gives information about first aid, medical treatment and rehabilitation after a heart attack.

This campaign has been followed up by a similar one which is jointly run by the HEC and DH called the Look After Your Heart (LAYH) programme. The immediate objective of the campaign is to increase public awareness and support for healthy lifestyles as a goal for all, with particular emphasis on contributing towards:

(i) a decline in smoking;
(ii) the adoption of healthier eating habits;
(iii) increased levels of participation in exercise by everyone;
(iv) a better understanding of the concept of 'stress' – what it is and how to cope with it.

The campaign will also be concerned with promoting general acceptance of:

(i) the need to avoid excessive alcohol consumption;
(ii) the value of occasional blood pressure checks;
(iii) the need to avoid obesity.

The longer-term aim is to seek to contribute to a downward trend in CHD and will complement the HEC's Heartbeat 2000 project.

The campaign is intended to be aimed at everyone although special focus will be on working-class groups. It focuses on direct communication with the public and will mainly take the form of a media campaign, production of suitable background material and extension of the Look After Yourself (LAY) campaigns. It will be supported by parallel efforts directed at the medical profession. After its launch in the spring of 1987, the campaign spent £15 million on three major fronts which were community-based activities, the role in industry and workplace, and the national mass media and promotional aspects.

An evaluation is taking place with an annual survey of public attitudes and publication of the Prevention Index. Results of the first evaluation of the mass media campaign show (McKenzie, 1988) that six months after the launch of the campaign slight favourable shifts in attitudes were recorded, particularly amongst working-class groups. Behaviour change was very small as might be expected given the type and duration of the programme.

The second phase of the programme started in the autumn of 1988 and particular emphasis is being placed on the development of the role of the primary health care team. The aim is to move on from increasing awareness of risk factors to attempting to modify attitudes and lifestyles in England.

This programme is part of HEC's longer-term strategy which has the following specific objectives.

Diet	to increase public awareness of evidence linking diet and CHD and to promote the recommendations of the COMA report on diet and cardiovascular disease (DHSS, 1984).
Hypertension	to increase public awareness of evidence linking raised blood pressure and CHD, to promote life-style changes moderating blood pressure, and to encourage the provision and uptake of screening.
Exercise	To increase public awareness of evidence linking exercise habits and CHD and to promote the uptake of regular physical activity.
Smoking	together with the HEC smoking education programme, to increase public awareness of evidence linking cigarette smoking and CHD, to promote non-smoking.
Stress	to increase public awareness of evidence linking stress and CHD and to promote techniques for avoiding or coping with stress.
Immediate care	to increase public awareness of the benefits of CPR and to promote CPR education.

It is difficult to assess how beneficial the HEC's campaigns have been because up until now results of the evaluation exercise have not been available. However, Farrant and Russell (1987), drawing on evidence from a qualitative investigation, suggested that the overall approach adopted in the HEC's programme was inappropriate and therefore ineffective. Farrant and Russell (1987) argued that the HEC's thinking was based almost entirely on the views and assumptions of middle-class professionals about working-class lives and failed to take into account the perceptions, values and interests of the target population. Farrant and Russell (1987) argue that this top-down approach misguidedly assumed that working-class people wanted short and simple messages which focus on the consensus elements in the evidence. On the contrary, they wanted more rather than less information and help to evaluate the conflicting evidence which was presented to them. Working-class people were sceptical of expert knowledge and were suspicious of commercial campaigns trying to sell the health message.

Farrant and Russell argue that the most appropriate approach would be a community development programme which builds on the ways that ordinary people see their health problems as perceptions of health. This cannot be divorced from other social and economic aspects of daily life. Such community development programmes are in existence (see Royston/Wardieburn Project, 1986) although there is still considerable uncertainty about how these programmes should be evaluated. A comprehensive community programme requires not only that the needs and interests of the population could be incorporated but that, coupled with information and activities, there should be a change in the social environment in which the population live. No such changes are recommended in the Look After Your Heart programme, although in the the Heartbeat Wales programme and in North Karelia attempts were made to change the environment by controlling tobacco advertising and increasing the availability of low-fat food products.

Thirdly, in recent government policy documents on the health service (Secretaries of State for Health Services, 1987) and on primary care (DHSS, 1989) general practice has been identified by the government as the policy solution to CHD prevention. Hence, the emphasis on incentives to provide clinics for preventive care and to provide advice to patients about different aspects of lifestyle (see Chapter 3).

WHAT SHOULD BE DONE?

Specific government policies aimed at preventing Coronary Heart Disease have been evaluated by a number of bodies but the most recent has been by the National Audit Office which is independent of the government (NAO, 1989). NAO's report has also been examined by the House of Commons Public Accounts Committee (HMSO, 1989). NAO's report examined both prevention and treatment services for CHD and the roles of the health department and the NHS in the reduction of CHD mortality and morbidity. In the area of prevention, the report suggests that policies have been hampered by the lack of a single study for co-ordinating government policy in the same way as for AIDS and drug and alcohol abuse. It also suggests that departmental guidance for health authorities in developing specific programmes has not been incorporated in national strategies hence the finding that there was an uneven approach to prevention amongst the districts. In addition, there was a lack of a comprehensive data base for morbidity and health indicators which hindered planning and evaluation. Also, the Regional Health Authorities provided insufficient information on local initiatives for the Department to assess the level of activity and for them to be integrated into the national campaign. Finally, the national programme in England directed at public information lacked quantifiable targets so it was difficult to assess its impact. Also, government departments and the NHS as employers have given little support to their programmes.

This report has in many respects been supported by the report from the House of Commons Public Accounts Committee (HMSO, 1989). Perhaps, one of the more significant conclusions which emerged from the report was this statement:

> We note the Department's admission that much remains to be done in heart disease prevention. We expect them to pay greater regard to the consensus view of the profession that a concerted effort by the health department and the National Health Service, supported by other government departments, is required to address properly the unacceptably high incidence of coronary heart disease in Great Britain.

CONCLUSION

The prevalence of cigarette smoking and the consumption of saturated fat has declined in the United Kingdom over the last decade, although there is little evidence of any reduction in the alcohol consumption or of a marked increase in exercise taken by the population as a whole. However, the prevalence of smoking, heavy drinking and consumption of fatty foods is highest amongst social classes IV and V (semi-skilled and unskilled occupations), whereas levels of exercise are lowest amongst that group.

Government policy in relation to the control of smoking, diet, alcohol and the encouragement of exercise has been characterised by a non-interventionist approach with the emphasis on persuasion and industrial self-regulation. Referring back to Beatties' framework in Figure 2.1, it is a paternalistic policy which has been based on authoritative knowledge and is inclined towards a more individualist orientation, particularly with the recent emphasis on the role of the general practitioner. The overall approach of the government has been described as piecemeal and many policy agencies have advocated a more interventionist role for the government. For example, there is evidence from other countries, particularly in relation to smoking control, that a more comprehensive programme, including direct legislation controlling tobacco advertising would have a much stronger impact on tobacco consumption.

Apart from the ideological position of the government itself, a number of barriers to legislation have been identified. One of these is the vested interests in the production and consumption of the product. Another is the confusion of interests in the government itself. Certainly, in areas such as smoking control, government intervention has tended to come in the form of fiscal policy rather than control of tobacco manufacture or promotion, mainly because it is easier for the government to use simple bureaucratic procedures for regulating tobacco consumption than entering into a more complex relationship to control production.

One area where the government is focusing its prevention initiatives is in general practice and the primary health care team. The second phase of the LAYH campaign is focusing on primary health care teams and the new government contract is trying to encourage general practitioners to have a greater involvement in preventive care. Thus, in current government thinking general practice appears to be the key policy solution for preventing CHD.

3 General practice and prevention

Policy analysis

In the previous chapter it became clear that the government's current policy solution for the prevention of coronary heart disease was to encourage greater involvement by the general practitioner and the primary health care team. Yet it would be misleading to suggest that this was a direction which general practitioners or their professional representatives did not favour. The first part of this chapter examines the recent professional development of general practice and shows how and why emphasis has been placed on a shift away from 'curative' care towards 'anticipatory' care. The second part focuses on some of the assumptions which underline current policy statements and the feasibility of general practitioners becoming more involved in prevention.

THE PROFESSIONAL DEVELOPMENT OF GENERAL PRACTICE

To understand the significance of the recent attempted shift towards increased involvement in prevention it is necessary to trace briefly the professional development of general practice. The structure and nature of general practice in the United Kingdom has been influenced by the professional aspirations of general practitioners themselves, their relationship with their rivals, the hospital doctors and allied occupational groups and their relationship with the state.

The control that hospital doctors gained over the medical market place in the nineteenth and early twentieth century set the agenda for future debates about the role of general practitioners and the identification of the most effective strategy for enhancing professional development. Should general practitioners follow the path of hospital specialists or should they try to create a distinct speciality of their own? In recent years, as we shall see, general practice in many respects appears to have opted for the second course of action.

This decision was informed by a recognition that specialised hospital doctors had made further progress in their professional development in the decade following the introduction of the NHS in 1948. At the same time, general practitioners had become an isolated and defensive group who had lost interest in challenging the dominance of hospital specialists. Their professional development was at a standstill and in many respects their poor conditions of work, low income, and long hours of work were the price they were paying for owning their own practice and being independent. Their position can be likened to the small shopkeeper and this approach has left its legacy in that in more recent proposals (Maynard, 1984; Enthoven, 1985) the general practitioner has been prescribed the role of the small-scale entrepreneur. In the decades after the creation of the NHS, however, the professional fortune of the generalists slowly began to change.

These changes began in some respect with the GP charter of 1965 which recommended that the methods of remuneration and terms of service of GPs be revised. The charter stemmed from a build-up of pressure for improved conditions of service from the profession, although one of the most obvious catalysts was the setting up of the College of General Practitioners in 1952. Certainly, the charter did result in a change in GPs' working conditions and there was a decline in the proportion of doctors in single-handed practice, a decrease in the amount of home visiting and a more extensive use of appointment systems and deputising services (Cartwright and Anderson, 1981). Similarly, Wilkin *et al.* (1987) report significant changes in the organisation of general practice in the years immediately after the charter's introduction.

> Between 1968 and 1975, 553 new health centres were opened in the UK and over 1,400 loans to convert and construct new premises were taken up. The trend towards larger practices continued so that the proportion of doctors in practices with three or more partners increased from 42% in 1964 to 60% in 1973. In the five years from 1968 to 1973 the number of wholetime equivalent clerical staff went up by 10% each year and the number of employed nurses by 26% overall. . . . A new concept of the primary health care team began to emerge.

Thus, in the mid 1970s, 25 years after the introduction of the National Health Service, general practitioners had gained control over their working conditions and created a distinct environment in which a profession could flourish. Not only that, but general practitioners had started to become employers and could assert their dominance over the primary health care team.

These changes, while improving the working conditions of the doctor, appear to have increased the social distance between doctor and patient by creating barriers between the two. This may account for the finding from Cartwright and Anderson's study (1981) examining changes in patient views about primary care between 1964 and 1977 which showed that despite marked changes in the organisation of general practice during this period, there was no indication of any greater understanding between doctors and patients. Indeed, from the patients' point of view, the quality of care they received had actually diminished in some respects.

While these organisational changes may have created further barriers between GP and patient the new specialist body of knowledge which the official representatives of GPs were trying to develop appeared to be aiming to bring the doctor and patient closer together. If further professional development was to be achieved, general practice appeared to require a distinct specialist body of knowledge, at least distinct from its rivals in the hospital. Up until this time GPs' professional aspirations were still modelled closely on hospital medical practice, reflecting the continuing dominance of the content and ideology of hospital medicine. For example, Armstrong (1979) has shown how problems or crises in general practice were defined through the perspective of the hospital paradigm, however inappropriate it may have been for a community-based service response to the demands of the public. The recurrent concern about trivial demands, the desire for hospital work, and the emphasis on academically acceptable foundations are all examples of the continuing influence exerted by the consultants over their generalist colleagues at this period.

About the same time, however, a different solution to the more traditional 'medical' approach was emerging from discussions initiated by the Royal College. This solution has been described by Armstrong (1979) as the biographic approach to medicine as it places emphasis on the need to consider the patient as a whole and to concentrate on the signs and symptoms in the context of the patient's own biography and environment. This holistic approach is represented in the work of Balint and Norell (1975) and appears to have been largely accepted by the profession's leaders, if the official pronouncements of the Royal College of General Practitioners (RCGP) are anything to go by.

The extent to which this model has been adopted at the expense of the traditional hospital-dominated model, is difficult to assess. However, results from a recent study (Calnan, 1988b) suggest that the GP population as a whole is split down the middle in that a large proportion support the clinical model and another large section support the 'holistic' model. One way that this evidence might be interpreted is that a clear difference is emerging between the world of the official representative of GPs and the world of everyday general practice. In some respects, the 'elitist' and 'radical' approach of the RCGP is becoming increasingly distant from the view of the majority of general practitioners. Yet, as Freidson has pointed out (1985) professional status does not hinge on the activities of an aggregate of individual general practitioners but on the activities of the profession's representatives. Hence, the 'holistic' model may perform the function of providing the profession with a distinct ideology which can be used at the official level even though it is not accepted by a large segment of working GPs. In some respects it merely acts as a political rhetoric.

Over the last decade or so, some of the developments which have affected hospital medicine have worked to the favour of the development of general practice. There is evidence of the growing popularity of general practice as a career choice for medical students in spite of the low esteem in which specialist teachers hold general practice. Between 1979 and 1984 GPs contracted for general medical service increased by 11 per cent from 26,000 to 29,000. This increase in popularity is probably due in part to the improved financial prospects of GPs and in part to relative freedom to practice medicine without the constraints of cash limits. Indeed, it is perhaps only in the last ten years that the independent contractor status of GPs has come to work in their favour when compared to the position of specialists. In addition, general practice may have become a more popular career option not so much because of its new 'holistic' model propagated by the RCGP but because of the failure of hospital specialist medicine to make progress. Certainly over the past couple of decades specialist medicine has seen relatively few major advances which have affected large numbers of people. The hospital-based specialists have made relatively little progress in dealing with the major chronic and life-threatening illnesses and this may have had the effect of raising the status of general practice compared with specialist medicine. In this respect, the cultural critique of scientific medicine has shaped doctors' perceptions as well as the public as a whole.

In some respects, then, this period saw an increase in the professional status of general practitioners which was further illustrated by the emergence of the debate about the content and quality of general practitioner care. The debate about the content of general practice focused on which areas GPs should expand into. It was shown previously that general practice as a whole was divided into those with a clinical approach and those with a more social orientation. This difference is reflected in the two distinctly different schools of thought which have emerged in the debate (Calnan, 1988b) about what broad areas of service general practitioners could be involved with.

The first school argues for a deepening involvement with clinical care, extending general practitioners' range of activities into areas such as minor surgery. One advocate of this position is the General Medical Services Committee of the British Medical Association (General Medical Services Committee, 1983) which argues that 'too many medical skills and aptitudes are laid to rest when doctors enter general practice. If general practitioners were given the opportunities and resources to use their wasted skills, it would result in a redistribution of work in the NHS'. Clearly, then, the concern is not just with creating a sounder base for the professional discipline but also with resource allocation and the money apparently saved if GPs rather than hospitals carry out certain medical treatments. This shows how broader developments in the health care system have implications for the professional development of GPs.

The other school of thought, rather than looking for a deepening involvement in clinical care, advocates shifting the focus and extending the GP's role into the area of health promotion and disease prevention. Much of the impetus for this change appears to have come from within general practice itself, although it clearly resonates with cultural and political discourses about healthy living and self help (Crawford, 1984).

GENERAL PRACTICE AND PREVENTION

While the major policy documents emphasising the role GPs might play in prevention emerged in the early 1980s there had been some debate about prevention before that. As early as 1950, a British Medical Association report portrayed GPs as specialising in continuous and preventative care, and in health education (Bond, 1950). A subsequent report of the General Practice Steering Committee argued that these specialisms should be seen as 'unique' and 'positive' features of a future general practice (BMJ, 1952).

In 1959 the College of General Practitioners set up a Working Party on the Relationship of General Practitioners with Hospitals and Preventive Medicine. For example, in a draft paper presented to the committee the following was stated about the role of the GP in health education.

> The family doctors should be the leaders in a national effort to re-assert popular opinion towards prevention of illness rather than cure of established disease. This effort should be planned carefully, and conducted at every level, with as much publicity impact as that attending the start of the NHS – with its emphasis on sickness. At the same time the family doctor must become the chief agent to effect the required change in public opinion. He must accept that his responsibilities are those of medical adviser to his patients, and that he should teach them how they may achieve health and remain well. The opportunity for health occurs at every consultation, when a patient willing to listen visits a doctor willing to teach. It is in individual in-service training, blended into the normal powers of diagnosis and therapy until it too becomes 'normal' that the doctor's strength lies. Teaching from the doctor's mouth is likely to be appreciated and accepted by his patients, and remembered when teaching from other sources has been forgotten. The advice given in the home is as valuable as that given in the surgery.
>
> (RCGP, 1959).

Interest in this area gained further momentum in the 1960s with the translation of the notion of continuity of care into a practical concern for early diagnosis (McWhinney, 1964) and with the re-definition of roles and boundaries within general practice that accompanied this (Jefferys and Sachs, 1988). Thus, by the 1970s a number of authors were pointing to the attributes of general practice which made it the 'natural setting' for health education (Calnan and Johnson, 1983) and were calling for an increased role in health education for general practitioners (Stott and Davis, 1979). Current interest in the role of GPs in health education stemmed largely from a series of reports produced by the Royal College of GPs between 1981 and 1983. In response to the publication on prevention from the Department of Health and Social Security in the mid-1970s, the RCGP set up its own Working Party to consider the issues in the interest of general practice. Five reports were eventually produced which looked at the role of GPs in prevention in general (RCGP, 1981a) and in four specific substantive areas (RCPG 1981b, c, d, and 1982). Whilst not constituting (policy) documents in the strictest sense, these reports were an attempt by the College to provide a clear statement of what it felt the field of interest should be in general practice.

In setting out the types of 'worthwhile preventive activities' of GPs the authors of the main report (RCGP, 1981a) delineated three main arenas in which they could be active. The first involved patients who present themselves in consultation. That is, with each patient who consults, the GP can extend the traditional content of the consultation to provide a preventive component. In addition to the prevention of complications of the presenting problem, the types of activities recommended include opportunistic screening for presymptomatic diagnosis of other problems and health education about lifestyle issues, particularly smoking.

The second arena is the practice population as a whole. Because each GP is responsible for a defined population of registered patients who may be divided into 'risk' groups according to age/sex characteristics (for example, men over 35) or medical criteria (for example, hypertensive, diabetics), he or she is in a position to monitor the health of such groups and to provide appropriate preventive interventions. This approach is seen as a radical innovation for general practice because it involves GPs in thinking in terms of groups at risk, taking the initiative in contacting them and co-operating more closely with other members of the primary health care team in providing the service. Once again, however, the focus is on personal preventive advice given to individual patients in the context of the one-to-one consultation.

The third arena, which is only briefly and tentatively described, is the local community. The GPs' responsibilities here involve working with professionals in other institutions in the community. A GP may, for example co-operate with school teachers in teaching about 'relationships', 'sexual love and childbirth', 'healthy living', 'preventing disease' and 'using the health services'. Aside from this example, however, little is said in the introductory report about the role of GPs in the community and it is seldom referred to in the subsequent reports.

Criticisms of this initiative from the Royal College of General Practitioners have been made on a number of levels; some have interpreted it as another example of the creeping medicalisation which is inherent in Western industrial society. It is argued that the medical profession – or one segment of it – is furthering its empire by attempting to claim justification over people's lifestyles, or those aspects of lifestyle which are claimed to influence disease. Others have suggested that the Royal College of General Practitioners' crusade in the area of prevention is a further attempt to maintain or enhance GPs' professional identity independent of hospital medicine. For example, as Honigsbaum (1985) states:

> They [the RCGP] fear most any move that will carry general practitioners closer to hospital medicine, so much so that it might be fair to describe their proposals as the 'keep general practitioners busy in the community' school. For them, almost any activity will do as long as it leaves general practitioners free from entanglement with consultants.

Honigsbaum also doubted the potential success of the RCGP drive since it focuses on education and changing expectations to involve GPs without any attempt to change the system of remunerations to reward their involvement in preventive activities. However, this criticism now needs to be modified given the recent proposed changes in remuneration in the new contract.

Others have criticised the RCGP's initiative because of the inherent individualism in its approach to disease prevention and health promotion (Davies, 1984). While the main report presents GPs as becoming involved in progressively wider arenas of activity, the view of their roles in each arena is in fact narrow and limited. The emphasis is almost exclusively on GPs dealing with individual patients in the one-to-one consultation. The kinds of issues which are discussed are therefore those which are best suited to personal advice in this setting: aspects of lifestyle and personal health choices. Broader issues of 'social conditions and standards of living' (RCGP, 1981a) are recognised as having a fundamental influence on health and illness but seem to be largely ignored as inappropriate or unrealistic topics in the context of general practice. Instead, in the aetiology of preventable disease the focus is on individual patients and their families whose behaviour is seen as the main factor that the GP can influence. The role of GPs, therefore, is restricted to that of educating patients and their families about personal health habits, and motivating them to change these when appropriate.

Implicit in this individualistic approach, which is inherent in health policy more generally in the UK, are two assumptions about the production on health and how it might be controlled (Graham, 1979). Firstly, the medical model of disease causation and disease management dominates as the emphasis is placed on individual causes which in this case are individual or family lifestyles. Secondly, the individuals are assumed to be able to control their own lifestyle and to be able significantly to improve their health in this way. Doubt has been cast on the validity of these two assumptions, which together constitute a form of 'victim-blaming' since the effect is to shift the responsibility for disease causation, cure and care away from broader socio-economic factors on to the individual who suffers ill-health (Labonté and Penfold, 1981).

More specifically, not only does evidence suggest that socio-economic factors influence patterns of lifestyle but it also suggests that there are other socio-economic influences on health outcomes which might be independent of lifestyles (Doyal, 1979; Townsend and Davidson, 1982). For example, social class differences in health status might be explained, at least in part, by the less favourable living and working conditions of manual workers which expose them to greater physical hazards. Moreover, the stress generated by financial problems, housing problems and problems associated with employment may contribute directly to higher rates of illness.

Additionally, recent empirical research has shown that there are strong barriers to the adoption of preferred health choices, particularly in conditions of socio-economic disadvantage. Many people are simply not in a position to alter their lifestyles or health decisions in response to GPs' advice and encouragement. Moreover, the relevance of 'good health' as defined in conventional health education terms might be of limited significance in some social circumstances where, for example, cigarette or alcohol consumption is based on rational rather than idiosyncratic premises. For women in particular, smoking and/or heavy drinking may be a rational way of coping with the pressures of living in conditions of social and economic adversity (Jacobsen, 1981).

On yet another level, further criticisms have been made of the RCGP's initiative because it ignores trends and patterns within general practice which may themselves undermine even the limited value of its individualistic approach. The first concerns the present organisation of general practice. If health education with the individual patient is to be effective, then relationships between doctors and patients need to be personal ones and their continuity needs to be maintained. At first sight these elements appear to be particularly strong in general practice. However, the development of group practices and the greater use of deputising services have led to an increasing impersonality and distance between general practitioner and patient. GPs are no longer the 'personal doctors' which it is often claimed they once were and patients may be less inclined to 'comply' readily with their advice. This loss of personal involvement on the part of GPs may be less of a problem if other members of the primary health care team were to become involved in personalised care but there is little evidence that this is happening.

A second set of criticisms concerns the variations in patterns of demand for general practice services and the variations in the quality of care given to certain groups. For example, for a complex set of reasons, women use general practitioners more than men, but the relative health 'risks' suggest that there needs to be a refocus on men (Townsend and Davidson, 1982). Similarly, there are cultural and sometimes racist barriers to help-seeking amongst ethnic minorities living in this country. Finally, there is evidence that working-class groups receive less medical information in general practice consultations from their middle-class counterparts (Pendleton and Bochner, 1980). Clearly, it is important to make health activities more accessible and relevant to the widely differing, and often neglected, needs of all groups within a multifarious society.

PREVENTION AND THE DOCTOR–PATIENT RELATIONSHIP

More specifically, there is the issue concerning the social organisation of the doctor–patient relationship and if the current structure is geared to effective communication the image of the general practitioners as health educators portrayed in recent policy statements is one where doctors help their patients to help 'themselves'. This form of relationship might be described as a mutual participation type and is thought to help maximise health education during the consultation. This type is characterised by doctors giving advice to help patients to help themselves and by patients becoming responsible for controlling their own health through the use of this knowledge and encouragement. In this instance, the general practitioner acts as a resource in matters of health and skills to help the patient change behaviour. The powers of the general practitioner and the patient in this relationship are viewed as being equal, although the basis of the two participants' power is different. The general practitioners' power comes from their more extensive knowledge of health and its control. The power of the patients derives from the fact that they ultimately decide whether or not to follow the advice.

Evidence from studies of doctor–patient relationships in general practice suggests that the mutual participation type of relationship is not common and that more often the relationship is characterised by a dominant and active doctor and a passive and dependent patient. This form of relationship tends to lead to a dominance of the doctor's perspective over that of the patient. This unequal relationship is said to be due, in part, to the difference in the level of knowledge of expertise between doctor and patient and to be maintained because of the lack of information given by the doctor to the patient. Certainly, one of the most common reasons for dissatisfaction with doctors is the lack of information given to patients about their complaints. Whatever the explanation is for this problem in the communication of information, the image of the doctor as health educator freely giving out information is not one which appears to have a realistic basis in empirical studies of doctor–patient relations. This form of doctor–patient relationship may be a product of the content of the consultation where the focus is usually on the diagnosis, treatment and management of illness and the relationship may change as a result of the practice of health education in the consultation. However, greater difficulties may arise if the general practitioner and the patient are so imbued with the curative approach that the practices used in an illness-orientated consultation are adopted in consultations where the general practitioner intends to provide health education.

Sociologists have also argued that the uncertainties in scientific medical knowledge influence doctors' behaviour in the consultation and are a potential source of tension in the doctor–patient relationship. In some areas, such as the relationship between lifestyle and health outcomes, it is claimed that uncertainties are particularly marked. By opening up the doctor–patient relationship into an equal partnership, the doctor may be open to criticism as patients become more aware of the uncertainties in scientific medical knowledge. This may lead to increasingly critical patients who may wish to change their general practitioners more frequently. It may also lead to doctors being increasingly reluctant to become involved in health education because of the considerable uncertainties in knowledge and the potential threat to their professional status. In addition, there is the question of how patients will handle these uncertainties in health knowledge. Studies of illness behaviour have shown that it is in situations of 'uncertainty' when sufferers and their families find they cannot explain their signs or symptoms, that decisions are made to consult medical practitioners.

Secondly, there is the question of how both general practitioners and patients make sense of the epidemiological evidence which might provide the 'scientific' base for the information which is given during the consultation. Certainly, in a study of lay health beliefs (see Chapter 5) perceptions of vulnerability to disease were rarely based on statistical models. The most common criterion for assessing vulnerability was whether there was a current or previous experience of signs and symptoms. Most abstract models were not common and feelings of vulnerability were rarely associated with personal behaviour.

The general practitioner as health educator also implies that the doctor should have an interest and knowledge of people's lifestyles, an understanding of why such lifestyles are adopted and how such lifestyles might be modified. Little evidence is available about general practitioners' concepts of health and illness, although those concepts

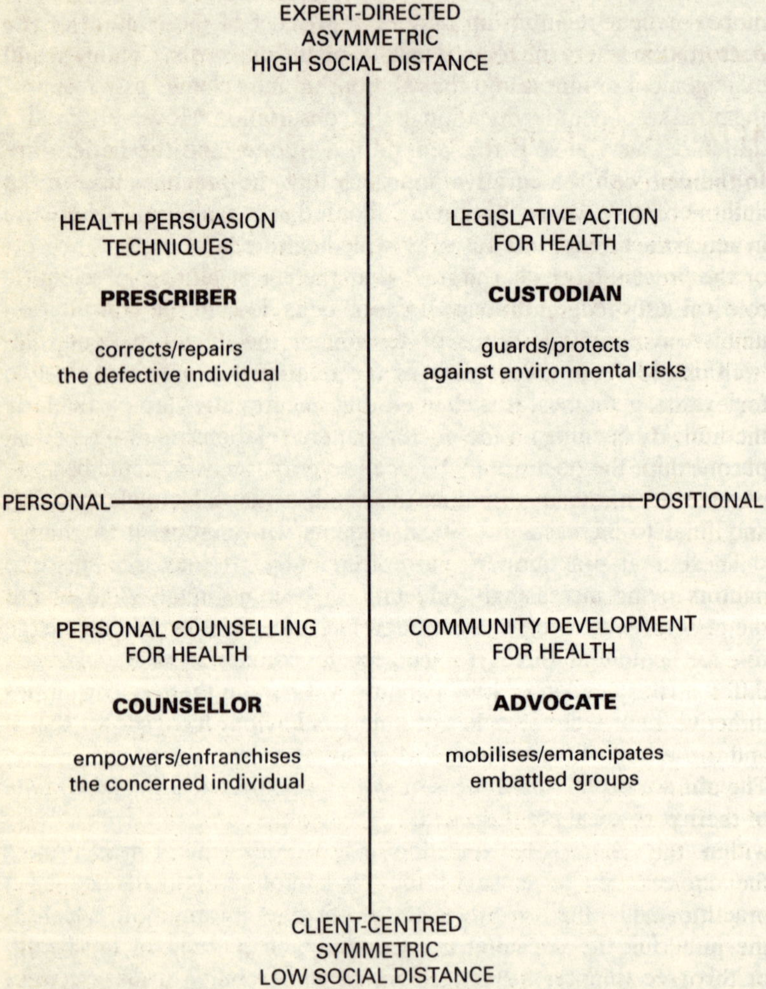

EXPERT-DIRECTED
ASYMMETRIC
HIGH SOCIAL DISTANCE

HEALTH PERSUASION TECHNIQUES

PRESCRIBER

corrects/repairs the defective individual

LEGISLATIVE ACTION FOR HEALTH

CUSTODIAN

guards/protects against environmental risks

PERSONAL — POSITIONAL

PERSONAL COUNSELLING FOR HEALTH

COUNSELLOR

empowers/enfranchises the concerned individual

COMMUNITY DEVELOPMENT FOR HEALTH

ADVOCATE

mobilises/emancipates embattled groups

CLIENT-CENTRED
SYMMETRIC
LOW SOCIAL DISTANCE

Figure 3.1 Re-casting professional roles in health promotion
Source: Beattie (1991)

of health which might be compatible with effective health education would place an emphasis on health as a positive state which must be understood within the context of an individual's social and physical environment.

Beattie (1991) in his analysis of the range of professional roles available in health promotion for doctors and nurses described them as shown in Figure 3.1.

The more conventional doctor–patient relationship falls into the area where doctors and nurses are prescribers and persuaders. The more recent depiction of the doctor–patient relationship is where the doctor is more a counsellor helping patients to develop themselves.

ALTERNATIVE ROLES FOR THE GP

In their preoccupation with the role of GPs in the consultation, the authors of the College reports give little attention to alternative ways in which they could be involved with their patients. Only in the report on the prevention of psychiatric disorders is mention made of a wider role for GPs. Here the sub-committee suggest that GPs are in a unique position to understand community needs and therefore are 'well placed to encourage community development' (RCGP, 1981b), for example, through patient participation groups. The criticisms of the individualistic approach reviewed above point to the importance of considering more carefully such alternative, collectivist approaches which can better take account of the broader issues involved in health and illness.

There are at least two strategies for health education within the nations of 'collectivism' which could have implications for the role of the general practitioner (Beattie, 1991). Both approaches identify a role for health education in encouraging social change although they differ in the degree to which the approach is directive. The more directive of the two strategies would involve general practitioners and the primary health care team in a public agenda-setting exercise. The aim would be for health professionals to increase the awareness of their patients and others in the local community about the forces within the social, economic and legal environment which limit the choices that individuals have in matters of health. General practitioners, therefore, might be involved in attempting to educate the public about the need to press for change through legislation or through other public policies. Such change, it is argued, would contribute towards the creation of a healthier environment per se, which would in turn enable people to adopt a 'healthy' lifestyle if they so chose. The drawbacks of this approach, however, are those inherent in all 'top-down' strategies of community action. That is, the models of illness causation and of appropriate intervention which dominate are likely to be those of the health professionals rather than those of the community which they are meant to serve. The pressures which are brought to bear are therefore likely to reflect the interests of health professionals and to perpetuate the effective disenfranchisement of the lay members of the community.

The second collectivist approach is less directive in that the emphasis is placed on ideas and issues generated by local groups and local people rather than on needs expressed by professionals. The role of the primary health care team in collaboration with other health professionals, such as Health Education Officers, would be to provide resources (skills, facilities, support, etc.) to local people to enable them to develop their own structures for effective action in meeting health needs. This approach, however, is also not without weaknesses. The recent proliferation of 'self-help groups', as one of the three categories within the community health movement (Watt, 1984), may appear as a positive response to local needs but these are seldom concerned with social change and many accept prevailing individualistic notions and medical models of health. Furthermore, there is a tendency towards over-reliance on 'volunteering', that is, the use of unpaid voluntary helpers, to tackle problems that should be the responsibility of the statutory services (Beattie, 1991; Watt 1984).

A number of community health development programmes have been put into action. A recent project in Scotland explored the development of health promotion in a deprived city area. A community worker was allocated to a primary health care team and specific sessions were allocated to a general practitioner to help develop the project. A range of health promotion activities were initiated which included practical activities, work with small groups and attempts to create structures for local concerns to be heard by decision-makers and service-providers. The project also shed light on some of the barriers to general practitioner involvement in community development projects, such as the rigid structure of their general practitioners' time with little flexibility for developing a community network of contacts and the short-term nature of their involvement. Those involved in community health education programmes also emphasise the need for evaluation of their programmes but argue that the more conventional behavioural model of evaluation is inappropriate. The emphasis in this community development approach on the need to base the programme on the ideas of the 'lay' public clearly suggests that the reactions of the client to the interventions should be seen as a crucial source of information for evaluation. However, there are others involved in the programmes whose ideas about appropriate outcomes may differ from those of the client. Thus, some advocate a pluralistic methodology which does not assume a consensus or agreement about one appropriate outcome measure but uses multiple outcome measures, each reflecting the interests of different groups.

Evaluations of community development programmes have focused on other dimensions in addition to outcome measures. For example, a recent evaluation of an alcohol education programme has focused on 'process' and has mapped out the social, cultural and political context in which the programme is being carried out. An examination of this context is necessary because these contextual factors are believed to influence the ability of the programme to achieve the desired impact.

GOVERNMENT, GENERAL PRACTICE AND PREVENTION

Up until 1950, the state had done more to encourage the professional development of the hospital doctors than general practitioners. During the 1960s, as we have seen, general practitioners managed to negotiate better terms of employment but it is only recently, since the mid 1980s, that the state has become more interested in general practice, and has started intervening between the producers and consumers of medical care to regulate and control aspects of general practice and consumer satisfaction. This is partly because it is seen as the key for controlling expenditure on health care. General practitioners are seen as important because they control access to the expensive hospital technologies and they could also provide a prevention service which is believed to be less expensive than curative care.

The state's increased interest in general practice is reflected in its involvement in vocational training which is now mandatory and the introduction of the limited list for prescribed medicines. Whilst the professional status of general practitioners was enhanced by making vocational training mandatory, there was vociferous opposition to the limited list both from the medical profession, including GPs, and the pharmaceutical industry. It is difficult to assess how far this has affected GPs' professional independence. Recent research on the effects of the limited list in general practice indicated that GPs generally have had relatively little difficulty finding suitable alternatives to black-listed drugs – the main problems being with cough medicines and multivitamins. On balance, the limited list has probably had more severe constraints on hospital specialists' clinical freedom than on GPs both in terms of restrictions on the patients they can treat and in terms of controls on prescribing, through policies such as generic substitution and the use of antibiotics.

The recent Green and White papers on primary care are also illustrative of the state's more active stance with regard to primary care. The White Paper (Secretaries of State for Health Services, 1987) which confirmed many of the proposals outlined in the Green Paper, had the following aims:

(a) make services more responsive to the consumer;
(b) raise standards of care;
(c) promote health and prevent illness;
(d) give patients the widest range of choice in obtaining high quality primary care services;
(e) give better value for money;
(f) enable clear priorities to be set for the family practitioner service in relation to the rest of the health service.

Raising standards of care and increasing involvement in health promotion were to be achieved by changing the means of remuneration; other policy recommendations included making 70 the compulsory retirement age, increasing financial support to improve practice premises, extending the role of nurses as prescribers, developing ways of giving consumers better information and a wider choice and providing financial incentives for vocational training.

Why has the state published these documents? As with the limited list, one reason is economic – the perceived need to get 'value for money' and to control the use of resources by linking it to performance. Care provided by general practitioners is also believed to be a less-expensive option than the ever-increasing costs of hospital-based high technological medicine, hence the recent focus on the problem of the 'referral' behaviour of general practitioners and the attempt to shift the care of certain types of patient from the hospital to the community.

There are also political factors to be taken into account. Evaluating the performance of GPs is in line with the state's policy of attempting to limit the autonomy of certain professional groups. The White Paper makes it clear that if GPs do not monitor the quality of their performance then they are at risk that the state will do it for them. Such a proposal of course appears to threaten professional autonomy and may be one of the reasons why the Royal College developed its Quality of Care Initiative in 1985. Alternatively, the emphasis on evaluation may be seen as another device for enhancing professional status through the use of scientific methods.

In addition, the plan to give nurses more responsibility for prescribing certain drugs is also in line with the state's attempt to restrict professional autonomy. In this case the strategy adopted challenges the profession's monopoly of certain skills on the grounds that the state is best equipped to decide how patients' needs should be met.

Third, and finally, there are important ideological forces at work. For instance, the White Paper's discussion of prevention would seem to reflect the state's current predilection for encouraging individual responsibility and self-care. Likewise, the recommendations for action on quality control and the need to increase patient choice is related to the state's attempts to promote consumer sovereignty in the market economy. The emphasis on individual responsibility is clearly illustrated in the following quotation from the 1987 White Paper (Secretaries of State for Health Services, 1987) on primary care:

> Much distress and suffering could be avoided if more members of the public took greater responsibility for looking after their own health. The government intended positively to encourage family doctors and primary health care teams to increase their contribution to the promotion of good health. These professional workers as well as dentists and pharmacists are in daily contact with large numbers of the public and represent the front line of health care; they are therefore very well placed to persuade individuals of the importance of protecting their health; of the simple steps needed to do so; and of accepting that prevention is indeed better than cure.

Thus, the White Paper outlines the government's intention to enter into discussions with the professions with a view to encouraging 'more health promotion sessions in general practice to advise and assist on, for example, prevention of heart disease, on how to give up smoking, and on diet'. More concretely, it plans to change financial remuneration to encourage health promotion. First, the payment of the practice allowance would depend on a doctor carrying out health promotion and prevention of ill-health activities. It states that 'when a patient seeks a consultation the doctor should take the opportunity to assess the patient's overall state of health and offer suitable advice. Doctors should also offer patients whom they have not seen for two years the opportunity to discuss ways in which they might continue to maintain good health.' More positively, the government aims to pay a special fee to encourage doctors to provide an initial clinical assessment (i.e. a health check and any necessary follow-up) for patients registering for the first time with an NHS doctor. In addition, it states:

> The government also intended to amend doctors' terms of service to clarify their role in the provision of health promotion services, and prevention of ill-health. Doctors will be encouraged to recognise the role played by other members of the primary health care team in meeting locally agreed targets.

In summary, the government's White Paper places an emphasis on expanding the role of the primary health care team in health promotion and disease prevention and makes particular reference to CHD prevention.

These proposals have been included in the new contract for general practitioners. In addition to the health promotion activities covered by the capitation fee, a new sessional fee is to be introduced for health promotion clinics. Clinics for which a fee will be payable include wellperson, diabetics, heart disease, anti-smoking, alcohol control, diet and stress management.

In summary, general practitioners' representatives have, as part of their drive for professional development, pushed for a shift away from curative care towards anticipatory care. This policy has been adopted by the government partly because of the political influence of the medical profession, partly because prevention in general practice is seen to be an inexpensive alternative to hospital medicine and partly because of its ideological approach which emphasises the importance of individual responsibility and self-care.

SPECIFIC POLICIES, EFFECTIVENESS AND INVOLVEMENT

More general policies about the role of the general practitioner in preventions were discussed in the previous section. This section describes in greater detail specific policies aimed at CHD prevention which have been proposed and implemented and assesses the evidence for their effectiveness. However, before these policies are outlined it might be useful to consider why general practice is considered as an appropriate setting for preventive programmes.

Prevention programmes for coronary heart disease in general practice can be organised by the practice itself such as screening programmes or clinics and can be carried out by individual general practitioners through opportunistic screening and health education during a consultation. An analysis of the relevant literature identifies many attributes of general practice that make it a suitable setting particularly for health education. The following list represents some of these attributes:

- The patient consulting the doctor expects advice
- Doctors are credible authorities
- Doctors are trusted by their patients
- People are in a more receptive frame of mind when they go to the general practitioner because they are anxious and they have more motivation to change their behaviour if they fear disease
- The general practitioner has a captive audience
- The general practitioner has frequent contact with patients
- The registered list of patients permits a systematic approach to local population screening and audited follow-up
- The general practitioner has unique access to manual worker groups which are at higher risk of diseases such as coronary heart disease
- General practitioners are working increasingly with the primary care team which includes health visitors who are responsible for some aspects of health education

Other bodies, while accepting the favourable attributes of the primary care setting, have set out specific proposals for the primary health care team. According to the Canterbury Report (HEC, 1984) important aspects of the teams' job are:

(i) raising people's awareness of health and the importance of lifestyle;
(ii) identifying and monitoring people at special risk;
(iii) taking a responsible attitude towards the community regarding the control of risks and treatment of related disease.

The report also makes the following proposals to support and enhance the preventive activities of the primary care team. Firstly there should be more overall planning for health promotion. Secondly, there should be greater awareness of the possible roles of many of the members of the Primary Health Care Team (PHCT) in health promotion. Thirdly, there is a need to develop links with the district health education unit. Fourthly, there is the need to detect and manage people at high risk. Fifthly, there is a need to improve records and information systems, and to develop professional education and training and research.

A more broad approach aimed at the identification and control of risk factors has been set out by the Royal College of General Practitioners in its report on the Prevention of Arterial Disease in General Practice (1981b). It suggested that the following programme should be applied to patients as they consult.

(i) Blood pressure testing. At least one measurement should be obtained from every patient consulting aged 20–64 every five years. Those with pressures 180/105 (diastolic phase 5, mean of three readings) should be offered treatment and followed up at intervals not exceeding four months. A threshold of 160/100 would be reasonable for those under 40 years of age.

(ii) Cigarette smoking. The smoking behaviour of all patients under 64 should be ascertained and recorded in terms of the average number of cigarettes smoked daily. Risks should be discussed in relation to family history and blood pressure. In patients who want to stop smoking plans for doing this should be worked out; these plans may include the spouse. Stopping smoking should generally take priority over the control of obesity, where these objectives are conflicting.

(iii) Obesity. All patients under 65 who look fat should be weighed and measured, and given a target weight within 10 per cent ideal weight-for-height. They should be advised on the risk of Coronary Heart Disease, diabetes and hypertension in relation to their family history. The aim should be a general shift in the mean weight-for-height of the whole population, rather than spectacular weight loss in a few very obese people. Simple education material on energy values of different foods should be given, contact offered with slimming groups, and reliable information should be made available.

The report also suggests that known diabetics, all women on oral contraceptives and patients maintained on thiazide diuretics should receive special attention.

The authors of the reports only expect some and not all of this programme to be implemented and suggest that an expansion of resources would be necessary for the full programme to be carried out. The expansion of resources which is recommended involves:

(i) the extension of the role of the health visitors into prevention in young and middle-aged adults;
(ii) the delegation of management of clinics available at ordinary consulting sessions and other times should be made to nurses;
(iii) more staff to keep record systems for invitation and recall;
(iv) increasing financial incentives or eradicating disincentives for general practitioners who undertake preventive work.

There have also been specific practical policies which aim to help GPs identify 'high-risk' groups. The best example is the creation of a risk score by Shaper *et al.* (1986) using data from the British Regional Heart Study. This was referred to briefly in Chapter 1 and the risk score (excluding serum total cholesterol concentration and electrocardiographic evidence) identified 53 per cent of CHD cases. The intention is for GPs to use this risk score on an opportunistic basis to identify people who may need appropriate medical care. Further evidence is needed to find out how feasible the use of this risk score is in everyday general practice and how effective it is.

Another example is the model for screening for risk factors set up by Jones *et al.* (1988). The screening programme focused on identification and treatment of risk factors in all patients aged 25–55 years in a general practice population. Patients were invited, by letter, to attend and their risk factor profile was estimated through information given on a questionnaire and through physical examination. The patients with risk factors were invited to attend a lifestyle intervention clinic organised by the practice nurses and then by the health visitors with the help of the local authority dietician. Of the 1,212 patients, 78 who were shown by screening to have a high cholesterol concentration experienced a drop in cholesterol concentration. The mean fall in cholesterol concentration in the 78 patients who showed a positive response to intervention was 1.1 mg/al.

Much of the total cost of the programme was offset by payment of items of service provided such as tetanus vaccine or cervical smears. Thus, the overall net cost of the study to a 10,000 patient practice was £3,500, or for the average 2,000 patients per doctor practice the net effective costs were £700 per partner.

Grace (1983) also assessed the cost and extra workload involved in running a screening clinic for risk factors for the development of coronary artery disease. He found that such a clinic generated a small additional workload (13 extra patients a month referred to doctor) and, allowing for the 70 per cent reimbursement for a nurse and the extra cervical smears it was possible to claim for, the net cost to the practice per month was small.

Effectiveness

There have been some studies which have examined the effectiveness of health education and screening. Most of the field trials in the area of health education have been on smoking (Calnan and Johnson, 1983; Fowler, 1986) and have particularly examined the impact of advice, leaflets and nicotine chewing gum. However evaluation is increasingly being applied to other areas such as leaflets about coping with stress (Kiely and McPherson, 1986). The studies have tended to concentrate on change in risk factors rather than longer-term outcomes such as changes in morbidity or mortality. The results show modest reductions in smoking behaviour in the short term and the problem appears to be one of maintaining abstinence rather than giving up initially (Calnan, 1982).

Even though these studies show only modest reductions in cigarette smoking, it must be emphasised that even modest changes might lead to considerable falls in the number of deaths from smoking-related disease. It must also be remembered that health education in general practice, unlike some elements of curative medicine, should be judged by changes in health outcomes in the long term and that it is unrealistic to place short-term targets too high.

The studies up until recently have mainly evaluated brief interventions given by general practitioners to smokers. A more recent study by Russell and colleagues (1988) has attempted to evaluate a district programme which consisted of the provision of a smokers' clinic which was set up to mobilise, support, and co-ordinate intervention by GPs and other health professionals in a health authority district. The aim was to see whether such a programme would produce a detectable decline in the prevalence of smoking in the whole community of the district. Of 27 practices (101 GPs) in inner London which took part in the study, 7 undertook a brief intervention with support from a smokers' clinic (SBI), 4 provided intervention without support (BI) and 16 acted as usual care controls. The estimated decline in self-reported smoking prevalence over the 30-month period following the start of the intervention was 5.5 per cent (from 36.4 per cent) in the SBI group compared with 2.1 per cent for BI and 2.9 per cent in the control groups (average). The decline in the SBI group was significantly greater than in the other groups which did not differ significantly between each other.

The brief intervention involved the doctors in noting the smoking habits of all adult patients attending their surgeries, advising all cigarette smokers to stop, giving them a leaflet about smoking and how to give it up, and offering nicotine chewing gum (on private prescription) to those who anticipated difficulty in stopping. Those who accepted the gum were also given a manufacturer's booklet explaining how it should be used. In the practices doing brief intervention (BI) without clinic support, the doctors recorded smoking status in their own handwriting in the patients' notes and received no ongoing support and backup from the smokers' clinic. The supported brief intervention (SBI) involved, in addition, the provision of special smoker/non-smoker labels for the patients' notes with space for follow-up attendances, a leaflet about the smokers' clinics available in the district, and reply-paid postal referral cards to the clinic of their choice, together with a series of five brightly coloured posters about the risks of smoking for use in the waiting rooms.

Results published earlier (Russell *et al.*, 1987) based on follow-up a year after the intervention provided some insight into why the SBI intervention was more beneficial. It showed that use of nicotine chewing gum was associated with higher self-reported success rates and general practitioners providing supported brief intervention encouraged not only more smokers to use the gum but also more effective use. The study also showed that only 45 per cent of general practitioners (on average) complied with the direction to record smoking status and when they did so significantly higher success rates were recorded. Thus, the authors conclude that better results might be obtained if general practitioners' compliance with the procedure could be improved and if they encouraged more of their patients to try nicotine chewing gum.

There have also been field trials evaluating the impact of screening for hypertension in general practice. For example, D'Souza *et al.* (1976) examined the impact of hypertension screening in general practice in a 7-year controlled trial. The evidence from this study indicated that although screening successfully identified new cases of hypertension, it failed to make any significant difference to the population blood pressure. Over 95 per cent of the new hypertensive patients discovered by the screening process in the control group had visited their general practitioners for some reason during the previous years. This suggests that 'case finding' by GPs would be more cost-effective than setting up separate blood pressure screening clinics.

There are a number of different projects which have been developed such as provisions of well-men clinics (Wrench and Irvine, 1984).

However, the project which has received the most attention is the Oxford Prevention of Heart Disease and Stroke Project. This project focuses on screening for risk factors, offering advice and treatment and training ancillary workers (eg a practice nurse) to do this. Receptionists and GPs encourage their patients aged 35–64 who consult to have a health check carried out by the practice nurse or health visitor. The nurse screens for risk factors and offers advice on how to manage health-related behaviour, or he or she may refer an individual to the doctor for treatment. Costs are largely reimbursible. A facilitator employed by the health authority co-ordinates this activity in a number of practices by offering information on systems for detecting and controlling high blood pressure, diabetes and smoking. Although there is no evaluation as yet of its effects on health-related behaviour, mortality and morbidity, there has been an assessment of the effectiveness of the role of facilitators in promoting screening programmes in primary care (Fullard *et al.*, 1987).

The results have shown that in practices where 'facilitators' provided support there was a doubling of blood pressure recording, a quadrupling of recording of smoking and a 5-fold increase in the recording of weight compared with control practices.

General practitioners and their involvement in CHD related activities

The previous sections described evidence which suggested programmes aimed at preventing CHD based in general practice might be both feasible and effective. But who provides such programmes and how prevalent are they?

Some studies have examined, if somewhat superficially, the involvement of general practitioners in smoking control and health education in general as well as in hypertension screening. In relation to health education, there is evidence (Jamrozik and Fowler, 1982) that, although most general practitioners confess an interest in health education, particularly about smoking, it is not in fact a priority for most of them during consultations (Fleming and Lawrence, 1981). For example, a recent national study (Calnan, 1988a) examining GPs' level of involvement in health education showed it was education about smoking and diet rather than that about alcohol or exercise or group health education which was the most popular. However, it is difficult to judge from this evidence what this involvement actually means in practical terms. It may only reflect GPs' enthusiasm for health education and confirm that in reality health education is rarely provided in any systematic way. For example, a study using observational methods (Boulton and Williams, 1983) found that GPs discussed smoking, diet and the use of alcohol in only a small proportion of consultations, including those in which the patients' presenting problems provided them with an opportunity to do so.

The documentation of GPs' involvement in hypertension screening is much greater than that for serum cholesterol. There are wide variations reported in the literature, ranging from 34 per cent in North East Scotland (Ritchie and Currie, 1983) to 95 per cent in the Thames Valley (Fleming and Lawrence, 1981). The finding in the national survey (Calnan, 1988a) showed that 34 per cent of the respondents indicated that they were 'very actively involved' and a further 30 per cent selected the next highest point on the scale. Overall, the great majority of these doctors (81 per cent) said that they carried out hypertension screening themselves, and only a small proportion (14 per cent) delegated it to a nurse member of the team. However, the higher the reported involvement, the less likely the respondents were to be carrying out the screening themselves.

Data from the national study (Calnan, 1988a) also showed that doctors were much more likely to be involved in the routine screening of men with a family history of high blood pressure or heart disease and women taking oral contraceptives than of men or women of any age who did not have these risk factors. The proportion of respondents routinely screening each of the categories of patients increased with their reported level of involvement in hypertension screening.

A review of four studies (National Forum for CHD Prevention, 1988) was carried out from 1981 to 1986 of 21,196 adult records held by 103 GPs who were in self-selected practices in that they all agreed to have their work scrutinised. The findings below show the ranges of group mean recording levels of risk factors for CHD in adults aged 25–64.

Blood pressure taken in past five years	25–65%
Cigarette smoking	22–50%
Weight	33%
Height	20%
Eating habits	7%
Exercise habits	3%
Occupation	42%

These figures suggest that even where GPs are willing to do the additional work to provide data, these measures of anticipatory care are very incomplete. However, Fleming and Lawrence (1981) organised GPs from 29 practices in the Oxford Regional Health Authority to audit random samples of their records for preventive measures and to discuss their results on a postgraduate education centre. Two-and-a-half years later, mean recording levels for blood pressure during the previous five years had risen from 53 per cent to 61 per cent and smoking information from 22 per cent to 30 per cent.

In summary, detailed information about the involvement of general practitioners in coronary heart disease prevention at the national level is not available. Local studies and studies based on self-selected samples suggest that giving advice about cigarette smoking and hypertension screening are the more common practices although information about what these activities involve is not available. Information on levels of serum cholesterol testing is almost non-existent.

Explanations for variations in involvement in activities aimed at CHD prevention is also difficult to answer given the lack of evidence. The small number of studies investigating the factors that influence variation in doctors' involvement in health education shows that doctors believe that one of the major barriers is the attitude of the patient. For example, an American study (Ford and Ford, 1983) showed that many doctors felt that people only seek health care and advice when they are sick. In addition, many doctors felt that the public holds health in low regard relative to other life values. A more recent study of trainee general practitioners in England (Boulton and Williams, 1986) showed that many felt patients were resistant and unco-operative in relation to doctors' advice. However, these studies also point to other barriers which have little to do with the patient. Some of these are circumstantial, such as the lack of time available for health education in the consultation, where priority is placed on diagnosis, treatment and prognosis. Other barriers are to do with the attitude of the doctor, who may doubt the value of health education and place more emphasis on the clinical side of medical practice rather than the social or behavioural.

Boulton and Williams (in Calnan *et al.*, 1987) also focused on the attitude to prevention and health education among 34 advisors and specifically on course organisers in two regions in South-East England. While not a 'typical' sample of GPs in the two regions, the approach used in this study manages to tie the way GPs defined health education to the types of problems and barriers that were perceived. They identified four different types of approach.

The first group, about a quarter of the sample, viewed health education as a new technical service to build into practice routines, for example, organising an effective screening programme and records checklist. They emphasised their role in promoting behaviour changes in individual patients, especially in relation to lifestyle and the use of the GP service. They did not discuss the acceptability of this kind of activity to patients but saw the constraints largely in terms of structural and situational factors such as practice management and the availability of appropriately motivated and trained staff.

These doctors stood in marked contrast to a second group (again about a quarter of the sample) which perceived health education in terms of the need to be 'responsive' to the patient's presenting problems. The emphasis in their approach was on 'explanation' which promotes understanding and helps the patient to cope and to make sensible choices. They showed considerable reservations about the more opportunistic forms of health education and prevention, in which the doctor's agenda assumes precedence over that of the patient. Accordingly, they were more likely to see health education on lifestyle issues as intrusive and moralising, as too narrowly physical and as beset by contradictions and uncertainties stemming from the epidemiological evidence on which it is based. Interestingly, it is this group which most often pointed to the important role of social (as opposed to individual) factors in the aetiology of disease and the constraints these impose on behaviour.

A third group of doctors (about a fifth of the sample) argued for an 'integrationist' approach. This would combine most aspects of a 'technical service' approach – which addresses longer-term behavioural outcomes – with one which meets the immediate needs of the patients in terms of explanation and understanding. Their rationale for this rested in particular on a notion of 'effective teamwork' and the application of new approaches to communication. It is members of this group who had been most influenced by the RCGP initiatives and who had most actively sought to develop policies for their own practices. Not surprisingly, they viewed the constraints on practising health education as emanating largely from doctors: in particular, from their erroneous perception of patients' expectations of doctors and of their lay views as barriers to understanding.

The final group (about a third of the sample) saw prevention and the doctor's role as health educator in more restricted terms. Health education was a part of their daily work but they defined it mainly in terms of problem-related interventions on smoking, weight and occasionally alcohol. Some participated in limited screening exercises, but few were willing to become involved in a more general promotion of health where this was apparently unrelated to the patient's presenting problem. In several instances this reflected a lack of knowledge of any of the recent RCGP initiatives on prevention. The purpose of explanation was seen largely in terms of achieving compliance. For these doctors, the disruptive effect of health education on the doctor-patient relationship and the 'resistance' of patients in terms of their lack of interest in and ability to understand medical issues, were seen as largely immutable barriers to effective health education by the the GP.

Others (Fullard *et al.*, 1987) have suggested that the problems lie mainly with the organisation of general practice and the following are the main obstacles for carrying out preventive activities; (i) the demand-oriented philosophy of general practice which leads to focusing on symptoms; (ii) the brevity of general practice consultation; (iii) the lack of a co-ordinated and systematic approach in daily work; and (iv) the failure to use the resources offered by the primary health care team.

Another study (Calnan 1988a), drawing on data from the national study in England and Wales, attempted to characterise those GPs and practices involved in a range of activities, including health education and hypertension screening. The study specifically looked at general practitioners' involvement in the provision of health education (smoking, alcohol, diet, exercise and health education to groups), screening services (cervical and hypertension) and minor surgical procedures (excising cysts, stitching cuts, taking blood and fitting IUDs). One aim of the analysis was to discover how widely these activities were distributed within the population of GPs as a whole. Were these activities randomly distributed and were they all carried out by the same group of GPs or are different GPs involved in different activities?

A clear pattern emerged from the statistical analysis of the interrelationships which showed a type of creeping specialisation taking place with general practitioners tending to provide one type of service at the exclusion of others. Thus, doctors appeared to cluster into three distinct groups. The first group was the health educators – those doctors who reported a high level of involvement in health education about diet, smoking, exercise, the use of alcohol, and (to a lesser extent) health education in the community. Those doctors also had a degree of involvement in hypertension screening, albeit less marked than their engagement in health education. The second group compares those doctors with a high level of involvement in the provision of services for women: cervical screening and the fitting of IUDs, and the third group consisted of the minor surgeons – those who reported a high level of involvement in excising cysts, stitching cuts and taking blood. Each group was separate and distinct in the sense that its active involvement in one area meant its lack of involvement in the other two.

The second part of the analysis attempted to see if it was possible to identify whether a distinctive type of doctor practising in a specific setting is associated with the provision of a certain type of service. The analysis showed that it was easier to characterise doctors who were involved either in providing minor surgical procedures or in providing services for women from those who reported that they were mostly involved in opportunistic health education. This might be explained by the fact that opportunistic health education in the consultation does not necessarily involve the doctor in allocating extra time or the use of special facilities and much will depend on the perspective of the doctor in terms of the value placed on health education. Hence, the findings in this study showed that opportunistic health educators tended to be more likely to add a social orientation to medicine as opposed to a medical orientation.

In contrast, hypertension screening was more likely to be carried out by older, female doctors who were trainers. It was also an activity which was more commonly found amongst general practitioners attached to larger practices.

In summary, there is more evidence about the barriers to involvement than about the level of involvement in CHD prevention-related activities. Some of these barriers appeared to be associated with the organisation and structure of general practice and others were associated with the perspective of the doctor which appeared to reflect, at least in part, the nature of medical training.

This chapter has shown how the current interest in prevention in general practice is a product of a number of different interests one of which is the concern of general practice to maintain a distinct professional identity. However, this approach is backed up by evidence that it is a feasible and cost-effective policy at least in the medium term. There is little evidence to show what the level of involvement of GPs in CHD-related activity is nationwide, although a number of obstacles to involvement have been identified.

So far the policy developments and approaches to CHD prevention have been analysed from the point of view of the 'expert outsiders'. But what of the perspectives of the key actors in this issue – the professionals themselves and the patients. These perspectives will be considered in the following chapters beginning with the perspective of the general practitioner.

4 The perspective of the general practitioner

It was shown in the previous chapter that the official representatives of the profession of general practice have, over the last decade, put a great emphasis on general practitioners and the primary health care team becoming more involved in preventive medicine, such as in activities aimed at coronary heart disease prevention. This chapter examines coronary heart disease from the perspective of the general practitioner and attempts to identify what the 'rank and file' of general practitioners think and do about the topic. Survey evidence from a number of studies in England and Wales investigating general practitioners' perspectives on a range of different issues including prevention (Mechanic, 1970; Cartwright and Anderson, 1981; Jefferys and Sachs, 1983) shows an overall enthusiasm for prevention and health education but a limited amount of actual involvement. Even where there is some reported involvement it is uncertain what the quality of the involvement is.

This chapter looks in-depth at what general practitioners think and do about coronary heart disease prevention. In particular, it examines the apparent discrepancy between what general practitioners say they would like to do and what they actually do. There is a dearth of detailed evidence which examines this issue and so the chapter draws heavily on a local study which was a small-scale investigation of GPs' beliefs and practices.

Tape-recorded interviews were carried out during the winter of 1988 with general practitioners who worked in the East Kent area. There was a mixture of both town-based and rural-based practices and practices with differing partnership sizes. Thirteen of the doctors were currently trainers and the remainder (6) did not have trainership status. Thus, much of the information was derived from a section of doctors who were probably more committed to general practice than most and who were aware of new ideas about general practice originating from the RCGP and other agencies.

The interviews were carried out by the author himself and a semi-structured interview schedule was used. The emphasis in the interviews was on trying to discover how activities related to CHD prevention were perceived, how much involvement the doctors felt they had in these activities and what were the obstacles to their involvement. Thus, the interview began with general questions about prevention and its meaning, followed by specific questions about the circumstances in which they identified and gave advice about conditions and behaviour associated with an increased risk of CHD such as smoking, alcohol, diet and weight, exercise and stress. The latter part of the interview dealt with questions specifically related to CHD prevention. It must be emphasised that this is an in-depth investigation using qualitative methods and aims to understand the nature of the general practitioner's approach to prevention. No claims are made about its representativeness. It is essentially descriptive and the small numbers do not require numerical categories to be presented.

The first few questions in the interviews focused on the doctors' views about prevention in general and whether it was a good idea, if there was anything that worried them about prevention and what obstacles there were to setting up a preventive programme.

VALUE ON PREVENTION

The vast majority of general practitioners felt that in principle prevention was a good idea. Phrases such as 'Yes, I think it has to be', 'I think that's logical and very sensible', 'prevention is better than cure' were used on a number of occasions, e.g. 'Oh yes, there is no doubt about it, you know the old adage of prevention is better than cure I think is a good one.'

While only one GP said he was not interested in prevention a number of others did voice difficulties with prevention although agreeing with the idea in principle. For example, one stated that the problem with prevention was not gaining immediate results:

> I suppose that the amount of work that you have to do in prevention may not necessarily give tangible and obvious results sometimes and it may be difficult to maintain one's enthusiasm for prevention, especially in a field like coronary artery disease where the factors

> are still debatable. . . . I am generally in favour of the principle as long as it can be kept in proportion as far as one's workload is concerned. You can only spread yourself around so much.

Another suggested that carrying out preventive programmes was easier said than done:

> I mean I get dozens and dozens of journals and virtually every journal contains some article saying GPs should know more about nutrition, GPs should know more about alcoholism, GPs are very poor about development assessment, GPs ought to do more preventive ischaemic heart disease and this sort of thing so whilst I among my colleagues recognised the devastating effect of CHD on the British population, whether in fact we are able, in our individual ways, to make much of an influence on it I really rather doubt because the pressures that we come under of increasing demands and expectations of the practice population do not leave us very much time to do as much health education, preventive medicine as we ought to be doing.

The reasons why the vast majority put such a value on prevention was not very clear although some did offer an explanation:

> Well, I suppose I have for 30 years dealt with people who have had them [heart attacks] and I think, poor old chap of 42, that is a bit harsh to have had a coronary and lost his job and you don't have to see too many of those before you say, 'well, I wonder if there is actually anything we can do about it'.

This idea about the harm caused by CHD particularly in younger people was articulated by a number of general practitioners who tended to put it in a wider context of prevention:

> I think you have got to look at what we do in ordinary day-to-day working [which] is picking up the bits where someone had got CHD or has a stroke or has some catastrophe and really it is a bit late. Therefore, it seems logical to go back, as far back along the stream as you can to pick up what you are able to pick up and do something about and I think one has got to look at a lot of factors probably far sooner in life than we do at the moment.

Some suggested that prevention might be a cheaper way of doing things:

> Costs – if you get rid of something which takes 40% of all deaths by doing something which costs say a miniscule amount compared

> with the overall cost that must be a good thing ultimately. If you talk about trying to improve the quality of life longevity is it a good thing or not, I don't know, perhaps one should already ask that question first, I think really, why should we all live longer really?

This question of longevity and the reasons for interfering with longevity was also referred to by a number of general practitioners who suggested that prevention needed to be put in a realistic context. For example, one stated:

> I really wouldn't be trying to prevent someone of 80 too much having a coronary. It's not a bad way of going. . . . We have all got to die of something and I think this gets forgotten.

In summary, the majority were enthusiastic about prevention mainly because it reduced suffering and premature death amongst younger people. However, some doubts were raised about prevention particularly about its value for older groups although these will be dealt with in the next section.

CONCERNS ABOUT PREVENTION

General practitioners expressed a number of general concerns that they had about prevention. Many of the concerns seemed to revolve around the response of the patient. A number doubted whether the majority of patients or the 'right' patients would use it. For example:

> Yes, it's often the people who really do need help who never [attend]. . . . I think a lot are frightened, a lot are anxious not to have their lifestyle disturbed in any way because they are comfortable as they are.

The second concern about the response of the patient was that the programme may inflate patients' anxiety and make them neurotic. For example:

> You can induce neurosis by bringing to attention problems which people haven't thought about before. You can induce anxiety needlessly. I think if you get a raised blood pressure it could be difficult to persuade people that it really isn't serious . . . raised blood pressure of any degree to the patient is horrendous. It may be high, normal or mild hypertension and to them it is high blood pressure whether they have got a diastolic of 120 or a diastolic of 95.

The third concern was related to the second in that some doctors doubted their right to intervene in their patients' lives. For example:

> the idea that you are interfering with someone who feels well and if you look at hypertensives . . . every time I diagnose someone I am conscious of the fact that they are probably going to have more time off work because of it. They are going to be coming down with other problems that they would no doubt have treated themselves at home when we are actually creating someone as a sick person when they have been feeling perfectly well so they then adapt to that role. I tell them they have got to come down for their blood pressure checks and I give them medicines and actually make them poorly in certain circumstances when they felt fit and healthy.

Other reasons were given which were not tied directly to patient response. One of these was the uncertainty about effectiveness. The second was the difficulties in carrying out prevention because of the lack of time and pressures of work. This was how one expressed his position:

> I am increasingly frustrated at the system in as much that because of the pressures on us, despite the drift downwards of actual practice list size, this is more than matched by the extended role that we are expected to play in so many ways so that unfortunately the extra time that we should be having to work in the preventive aspect of medicine, is increasingly being absorbed in things like the emotional side of unemployment and the high incidence of marital breakdown, and the fact that there is no religion in society so that we are required to pick up all the social and psychological problems.

The third was to do with the priority which should be placed on prevention. One GP suggested that curative medicine should take priority:

> It would worry me if it [prevention] became all consuming, particularly in country general practice, and this is what we try and teach our trainees first, the first aim is to produce a safe doctor not necessarily a very good one, but a safe one . . . that means he doesn't miss too many of the big medical and surgical emergencies.

Fourth, it was implied that too much might be expected of a preventive approach:

> I think sometimes people's expectations can be raised too much by

> all these preventive measures all these clinics and things like this that it will keep them healthy, maybe too much of our resources will be diverted into it. The other thing is, can we afford to run preventative medicine to the degree that it's being pushed at the moment, like the cervical cytology services would be totally swamped.

Finally, there was the GP who felt that his role in preventive medicine has been over-emphasised:

> I think we ought to be bringing people up in schools and at home to look after their health better than they do at the moment. I am sure GPs have a role in that but there are an awful lot of people who are perhaps more important than we are who should be getting the right messages across because what we're talking about is trying to correct people's bad habits and I prefer them not to have the bad habits in the first place.

OBSTACLES TO PREVENTION

Some of the concerns about prevention were also evident when general practitioners discussed the actual and possible obstacles to prevention. For example, one obstacle which was referred to by three doctors was gaining enough enthusiasm amongst their patients to get a high rate of uptake. However, by far the most common obstacle was the lack of time as the following example clearly illustrates:

> The obvious one [obstacle] and the one that always crops up is time, finding the time to do it. I tend personally to feel that it shouldn't be a big problem because it should be a rewarding experience. We tend to find that if I have a lot of good ideas in the practice then it either means we are doing a lot of extra work or they don't get done but that is what happens in general but I haven't done anything because I haven't wanted to personally commit all the extra time to it [prevention] so at the moment we are stepping down slightly and suggesting that our practice nursing sister runs a well man's clinic of sorts.

Some doctors felt that because of this heavy workload there needed to be some kind of financial incentive to get doctors to put a priority on prevention. For example:

> It is all very well saying you should organise a system whereby you send for all your middle-aged men and check their blood pressure. No one pays our postcards or our stamps. We do get a bit of reimbursement on our secretarial time . . . as it is we have a very aggressive cervical smear policy and that for the practice is really quite an expensive exercise.

Other organisational elements were also referred to such as the lack of a computerised age/sex register and, as the following doctor stated:

> Organisation, I think. It's having the will to organise your practice in order to sort out your people to be screened that is you have got to build up your own age/sex register first whether it is manual or computerised. Then you have got to have the will to go through that age/sex register and to send out [letters], I mean, there are other ways of screening but if you are going to try to cover everybody, you have got to do it on that sort of basis. So you have got to have the will, the organisation and finance.

CONCEPTS OF PREVENTION

During the course of general practitioners' discussions of their views about the value of prevention, their concerns about prevention and the obstacles to the development of a preventive programme, their ideas and concepts about what prevention was or what it involved actually emerged from their accounts. It must, however, be stated that these concepts were explained in the context of an interview about the prevention of coronary heart disease.

The concept of prevention which tended to be the most popular and most prevalent was one which identified prevention as involving screening and/or advice-giving about lifestyle such as smoking and drinking. Involvement in prevention appeared for many to be the provision of well woman clinics or well man clinics although opportunistic screening was also mentioned. Opportunistic advice-giving was also mentioned frequently particularly in relation to smoking. Concern was expressed about the preventive programmes for the patient population as a whole rather than just those who attended the surgery. Certainly, the 'problem' of patient uptake appeared to be a major issue for general practitioners.

Taking blood pressure

The interview then focused on more specific activities which had implications for CHD prevention, if in some cases only indirectly. However, the activities were not discussed directly in relation to CHD as many of them were associated with other diseases or health problems and thus could be carried out for reasons other than CHD prevention. The first of these activities was the taking of blood pressure.

The most common circumstances, perhaps not surprisingly, under which blood pressure was taken was during the consultation. Although some practices were providing well person clinics where patients could arrange an appointment to attend or walk in only one doctor said that he had a system for sending out invitations for patients aged between 35 and 65. He stated:

> We also have a small screening procedure for patients between 35 and 65, their notes are checked, if they haven't had a normal blood pressure check in the last five years then a letter goes out to have their blood pressure checked.

However, the doctor also stated the system wasn't very successful because of the low uptake. This was also a problem which was found with walk-in clinics. For example, as one doctor stated:

> We have a well-person's screening programme whereby anyone who wants a checkup can come at their own convenience and see the nurse or the doctor where their blood pressure is routinely checked. However, the highly motivated health conscious ones will tend to make use of that and the other ones who most need it, won't.

The problem of low uptake or the wrong person attending seemed to be based on the doctor's own investigation of the results although it might also be a part of conventional rhetoric.

There was some routine screening of certain groups such as pregnant women and women on the pill through the consultation, assuming that both these groups will have attended their general practitioners. In many practices new patients routinely had their blood pressure taken as part of a general examination. However, apart from these groups the policy of routine screening becomes rather haphazard. A number said that they attempted to take the blood pressure of anyone (usually young adults onwards but some were aware of the need to take the blood pressure of children) who hadn't a recent record of their blood pressure taken. Sometimes this was in the past five years and for others it was in the past year. However, the actual implementation of this policy was rarely systematic and it was suggested that the full implementation of this policy depends on the level of work.

> Normally, unless there is a great pressure on time, I will do it if it hasn't been done fairly recently. So, if they have had a normal blood pressure in the last year I wouldn't do it but if I haven't got a normal value written down in the last year and there is time I will check it whenever I can . . . probably not for children but for all adults . . . except there is one group that we always miss out and those are the people who only ever come when there is something gone actually wrong and they never make an appointment so they are always the ones when there is never time to do all the routine things that you may like to do.

Most doctors tend to use this general approach combined with policies for specific groups of patients with certain clinical signs. Others tended to confine themselves to certain types of patient. For example, as the following doctor points out, this can involve consideration of a range of different patients.

> We check blood pressures on people who are on blood pressure medication and the routine review is normally three-monthly and is usually carried out by the doctor but sometimes by the nurse depending on the patient's preferences . . . if a patient has a symptom which could be related to the cardiovascular system then almost certainly I would check their blood pressure. If they had any other disease, say they came in and complained of weight loss or irritability or depression or something like that then I would probably do it. I think in those sort of situations I do it because it is expected of me rather than I feel I need to do it.

Others were more specific about signs and symptoms.

> A young fit healthy bloke who hasn't got any symptoms I would not start taking his blood pressure – but I would take the blood pressure of any diabetic, [anyone with] urinary troubles, anybody under stress, [or with] headaches, nose bleeds, etc.

All the doctors said that they tended to take both diastolic and systolic blood pressure and record them both in the patient's notes. Diastolic pressure was the measure the majority of GPs went by to assess elevated blood pressure although some were aware that there was increasing interest in the systolic measure.

Many of the GPs were also aware of the need to take more than one blood pressure measure if an elevated blood pressure was identified. For example, one stated:

> We take two blood pressures and an average . . . if the nurse finds an abnormal blood pressure then she will refer to one of our routine clinics. The doctor will re-check and then it would depend on a number of factors, it depends on the doctor's attitude to hypertension; it would depend on the level of the reading mostly, if the doctor finds it raised, he will bring them back in two or three weeks and see them a number of times before actually initiating treatment. Blood pressure tends to come down progressively with progressive readings.

Some doctors talked more broadly about elevated blood pressure and how it was defined. For example, one stated:

> There is no line because of course one's blood pressure increases as one gets older. We tend to go by the diastolic pressure rather than the systolic pressure and the diastolic pressure is normally in the region of 80 to 85 in the normal young adult and it creeps up throughout life so that the blood pressure of 100 diastolic or even 105 in an old person is quite acceptable so you do it really by age as well as by height. The significance of the systolic blood pressure I am not sure about. Up until recently we were told that this was not important, it was only the diastolic pressure that mattered. Nowadays people are a little bit more interested in the systolic pressure in that if it was very high they want to bring it down a bit.

This doctor also remarked on the patients' perspective about blood pressure.

> No, patients don't know what their own blood pressure is . . . in actual fact patients, particularly when you are treating them, they feel worse when their blood pressure is low than when it is high and this is one of the barriers to treatment and they say those pills disagreed with me. This is simply to bring their blood pressure down and you have to be a bit cautious about treatment not to lower the blood pressure too fast or they will opt out of treatment. The person who comes in and says, 'I know my blood pressure is high today' and is often quite wrong.

In summary, the vast majority of general practitioners clearly placed a value on blood pressure taking and many of them would have liked to take it routinely on all the patients who consulted. However, the routine taking of blood pressure, apart from women on the pill and pregnant women, was rare and tended to occur on self-selected samples of patients who attended well-person clinics. Blood pressure tended to be taken on those with clinical signs which were general and specifically related to cardiovascular disease. Opportunistic blood pressure taking was therefore widespread although in the main it tended to be initiated by the type of condition being presented and sometimes patient demand. The need to take more than one blood pressure was widely accepted when the blood pressure was elevated. Diastolic pressure was primarily used as the indicator although both were measured and both were recorded in the notes.

Advice about smoking

The second specific area of interest was smoking and the doctors were initially asked about how they identify smokers.

Identifying smokers

Apart from the people attending well-person clinics, the only others who were asked about their smoking habits, regardless of clinical signs and symptoms, were new patients.

> I enquire about every new patient that I meet whether he smokes as part of a routine run through that takes just a few seconds . . . every time I meet a new patient I have never met before I ask them to give 30 seconds worth of their previous history, allergies, drugs they are on, whether they smoke, whether they drink, what job they do and who else is in the family and that really does only take about 30 seconds. . . . I have always done this for my new patients although the turnover in the practice is not very great and so there is probably an awful lot that I don't know about but I also ask everybody who has any symptoms that might be caused by smoking. If our computer system worked there is a little box there for recording smoking and so in theory we should know about an awful lot of them, in fact we don't.

The need to record smoking for the sake of insurance was also a frequent reason given. The vast majority of circumstances during the consultation when smoking was referred to involved a response to conditions although the range of conditions varied considerably.

For example, here is a general practitioner who offers a broad approach:

> Theoretically almost any situation and anybody coming in about the age of ten upwards one should really ask, in practice it's mainly people with angina, chest problems, coronary problems. I don't know that I always ask antenatal but, yes, in theory you should do. Certainly anything related to the heart, lungs or circulation.

Others said they tended to restrict asking about smoking to specific signs and symptoms. For example:

> Similar sort of things really [with] new patients and when people present with heart troubles or a cough or 'flu or something like that you ask as part of your knowledge of the patient . . . if it looks as though someone is coming in with recurrent bouts of coughing and spluttering and they are coughing and smell of smoke then I want to know whether they smoke. However, with a sprained ankle I wouldn't.

In summary, then, smoking tended to be identified either when a patient was newly registering or for a range of signs or symptoms associated with smoking-related disease. The range of signs and symptoms was varied although some tended to tie smoking practices up with other preventive procedures such as blood pressure testing. The overall impression was that smoking was high on the doctor's agenda and the majority felt that it was necessary to identify those who are smokers.

Advice-giving

Almost all the doctors had a reasonably well-thought out policy for advising against smoking. There were, however, some exceptions, as the following extract illustrates:

> Not being a smoker myself I tend to forget that other people smoke and that I should be a bit more aggressive about it. . . . I haven't got into the habit of doing it and I think that is my shortcoming.

The remainder seemed to have a well-defined policy ranging from instructional and interventionist strategies to straightforward education and assistance. Obviously, many individual general practitioners fell somewhere in between although the majority tended to err on the side of being instructional. Here is an example of those who only felt that they should educate:

> I would suggest that they cut down their smoking and that's all, it's their business, it's not a crime. . . . We have got some out there I just talk to them and say, you are smoking too much or something like that but then they will see me having the odd cigar in the pub you see, this is what I mean about the country practice doctor. . . . I have given my advice, we are only here to give patients advice, thank God we are not in a position to make people change.

The direct approach was used by many doctors although their approaches varied considerably. For example, one described his approach although this was influenced by his feelings about the effectiveness of the advice:

> Well, over the years I have become thoroughly demoralised at the effect that the advice that I give to patients on smoking has had. In other words, I don't know if I ever influenced people to give up smoking. I suspect I do to some extent but compared to the actual amount of time that I spend talking to patients about it [it] may be as minimal effect. . . . Yes, what I usually say is it looks like you probably have angina, tell me do you smoke? Yes, 15 or 20 a day. I say, my God, you must be mad or something like that and I write very pointedly in the margin of the notes, sometimes in red ink, 'smokes 15 to 20 a day,' Yes, so I tend to go nowadays I think for the short sharp emotive sort of response rather than the long intellectual discourse on the problem. If when they come back they are still smoking as much, I adopt the defeatist approach. I say 'well look I am not going to waste my time telling you how dangerous this is, it's your life, I will see you in the coronary care unit', or something like that. I really have got tough, in fact I say to people sometimes, 'look I am not going to bore you with talking any more, it's up to you.' The other one I sometimes use is, 'I suspect that smoking is far more harmful than we are actually told' and that I believe that it is a political thing that there is so much money involved in a political sense, that all we are allowed is a little bit of information from time to time. Now whether this is the truth or not I really don't know that.

This doctor clearly had an elaborate strategy for advising smokers and tended to use an aggressive approach. Others, similarly, offered an interventionist approach but were aware of the possible dangers.

> No, I put my cards on the table to start with and I admit to them that I am anti-smoking and that I feel that everybody should stop smoking and then I tell them why in their particular case I think it is particularly appropriate for them because I have got a bit of a reputation locally. Some people with chest infections choose not to see me because they know I am going to stop their smoking and they will go to my partners because they didn't want to be nagged by me. So I always start off by saying that I am against smoking and that although I do tell everybody to stop smoking I feel that it is particularly irrelevant for them because people were coming and saying, it's no good for you telling me to stop smoking, you just say that to everyone and since the impact was lost.

The fear that their patients avoid them because of 'bullying' about smoking was expressed by a number of general practitioners. They also suggested that their policy varied according to the type of smoker, i.e. motivated/non-motivated; old/young.

Leaflets, advice and referral to clinics were some of the strategies used by doctors although their approach tended to vary with the motivated, unmotivated, and old and young. Other strategies used were referral for hypnosis, acupuncture, or the prescription of nicotine chewing gum. Some felt the problem lay with motivation:

> Will-power is the only one, isn't it? Being scared. A patient came in with a bad cough and he looked very much like he was going to have lung cancer and we had the chest x-rayed and it turned out that he didn't have but that put the fear of God into him and he has stopped smoking and he needed something like that.

Finally, the majority of the general practitioners, as some of the examples have already illustrated, had doubts or were uncertain whether their advice giving and other interventions were effective. Much depends upon the level of motivation or the doctor–patient relationship.

> Again I think it does depend to a certain extent on rapport in the doctor–patient relationship. If you have got a good rapport they will toe the line hopefully a bit more than those with whom one doesn't have that support.

The idea that some people didn't want to hear was reiterated by a number of general practitioners and is well illustrated in one doctor's advice to pregnant women attending antenatal classes.

> I mean I have spent this morning in the antenatal clinic and I have tried very hard on three people. . . . There is a very clear relationship between smoking and small babies. . . . On the whole it doesn't work. They have already decided you see, they decided to give up smoking prior to getting pregnant or they decided, it didn't hurt me I don't believe what the doctor says, damn it. I am not going to listen anyway . . . these particular types of patients are of lower social class and tend to be less intelligent.

Certainly, there was great scepticism about effectiveness, although many didn't seem to know because they hadn't asked:

> I would like it to be effective. I am not sure that I would stop giving it even if it wasn't effective, especially being a reformed smoker. It would be interesting to do a survey and see how effective it really was, but having read reports on how to stop smoking it seems a good talking to by the doctor is in fact relatively effective.

Others doubted whether they could or should have that much influence.

> Yes, sometimes it is effective . . . you like to think so but it boils down to yourself, no matter what doctors say, for God's sake, people see adverts on the telly, they all know the risks you can expect, although some doctors think they are great, you can't expect to have that much influence on people until they have decided themselves to stop smoking.

The recording of smoking in the notes seemed to be variable rather than routine. New patients smoking seemed to be recorded routinely and many of the GPs said that they usually recorded it when they identified a smoker. Around five said that they didn't usually record it or only when the patient had reported giving up. Others emphasised smoking in the notes by ringing it with a red pencil.

Advice about alcohol use

While identification of smokers and advice about ways of controlling smoking seemed to be firmly on the agenda, for the majority of general practitioners identification of and advice about alcohol use appeared to be a low priority. Apart from the routine of asking a new patient, identification of a heavy drinker tended to be a rare occurrence related to certain symptoms or signs. For example, this was how one GP described his approach to drinking:

> [I enquire about alcohol] much less often than I do about smoking. Again if it is a new patient I will probably ask in passing but might forget to and unless they have got some sort of obvious related problem or they look like a boozer or I have heard through their family that they are a boozer and they have primed me to ask. You get the wife coming saying when he comes in next week could you ask him about his boozing, but we all know alcoholics are notoriously secret and again it's up to a person's common sense and I feel really one is on a hiding to nothing to stop a true alcoholic. It seems to be an absolute waste of time.

The point that patients tend to under-report their drinking was mentioned by many doctors and was used as an example of the difficulties in this area. Some tended to respond where there is only clear evidence, such as the smell of alcohol on their breath, or would use a more subtle form of detection:

> It's particularly difficult because when you suspect that they have a drinking problem you almost invariably get a brush-off. They say, oh no, I just have a couple of beers or something and you know full well it's a damn lie. Again, one tends to ask them more directly when there is something to suggest that there is a drink problem or when they have got something that has clearly been related like a duodenal ulcer. One of the findings that alerts one's mind to it is when you prescribe something for the patient and they say, is it all right if I have a drink with it. Then you know that drink is important to him and that really alerts oneself to the fact that they carry on drinking.

Why then do general practitioners rarely investigate the drinking habits of their patients? It is difficult to tell apart from the evidence that GPs find drinkers difficult to elicit information from and probably difficult to handle. Apart from the obvious signs (smelling alcohol on the breath) there seemed little awareness about the type of illnesses that could be used as clues. There also seemed a generally low level of motivation as the following extract suggests:

> I think because it is a much bigger grey area with alcohol consumption in that most of us drink alcohol at sometime, unlike smoking you are either a non-smoker or a smoker so there is a large grey area where GPs are not sure whether the amount their patient is drinking is excessive or whether they compare it to their own alcohol consumption.

The strategies for dealing with heavy drinkers were varied although much depended on identification and definition of drinking problems. For example, some GPs focused on what they described as 'alcoholics.'

> I think that if you have got somebody [who is at] the stage of becoming an alcoholic your prognosis is probably poor, much worse than [for a] smoker. One talks to them, tells them what you think the problem is, suggest the AA but with the feeling that you are very unlikely to get anywhere . . . obesity, smoking or alcohol there is just this feeling and you feel your heart sort of plummeting when it comes out because you feel so useless.

Clearly, this doctor was sceptical about the value of his efforts at influencing the drinking habits of some of his patients. Other doctors defined drinking problems more specifically:

> Anybody over 21 units a week may well be heading for trouble and this is quite a reasonable level of drinking I might say . . . I mean that is three units a day, a pint and half a day or three wines or three scotches or whatever and that is over a week and you will find that somebody can drink that in an evening or half a day but it is something to hang their hat on . . . it makes them go away and think about it that's all. I am trying to make them think about it really to start with. If you are dogmatic with people my experience is . . . particularly with alcoholics or anybody who is heading in that direction is that you have got to get them on your side to start with and they will come back when they really need you. They may not be ready for it that minute but in six months or a year they will say I have got to do something about it.

Many general practitioners, once they had identified the problem, gave their patients the option of referring themselves to AA or a specialist centre:

> If there is someone whose life is being ruined by drinking then we will offer them referral to AA or the Alcoholic Unit at A or even better to B which is a private mental hospital with a quite separate alcoholic unit further away if they can afford it that really is good. Yes, go for about three or four weeks but it costs.

Finally, it became clear from many of the transcripts that one of the most difficult parts of the 'treatment' process was the initial recognition of the 'problem' by the patient. Certainly, there was also a belief that the responsibility for ensuring the effectiveness of the treatment lies with the patient and the patient's general approach. For example:

> Well the first thing of course is to try and get the patient to recognise that they have got a drink problem and I think that really is the difficult one. I mean if someone hasn't got much of a drink problem then they are going to say, oh that's all right I can manage to give it up, it's no great thing as far as I am concerned and they appear to be honest about it. When there is a drink problem then they won't admit it. It seems to be a natural part of an alcoholic to vehemently deny there is any problem.

Alcoholics were then seen as trouble and, as the following doctor pointed out, were given a low priority:

> If they show willingness to be treated then we can offer to see them on a regular basis to give them some moral support or refer them to Mt Zion which is an alcohol unit which required a bit of travelling to, so they have got to be motivated for that but I think we have all discovered that we don't have a great deal of success in persuading an alcoholic not to be an alcoholic unless again they want to stop being one and I quite quickly give up on them.

While identification of drinking habits was much less frequent than smoking so recording in the notes was also irregular. For example:

> I think if one has considered it relevant to ask about drinking then yes one would probably write in the notes but not an awful lot of people get asked so I think you would have to go through a lot of notes before you find one.

Identifying dietary problems

Being overweight was the common criterion that almost all the general practitioners said was the major indicator of someone with a diet-related problem. It wasn't clear from the doctors' accounts, however, what was meant by obesity, although the following GP was the most specific of the group that were interviewed.

> Well, the obvious one is if the person is grossly overweight and having trouble getting around, out of breath, out of sorts . . . another thing would be a cardiac related thing, gastric related condition, anything that might I felt be related to a diet that wasn't right.

Other doctors said that it was a matter of judgement and how patients' weight had changed over the period that they knew them.

> You can see whether they are overweight or not you really don't need scales you just see a guy coming in with a bit of a pot on his tummy or the [woman] who you knew as a slimline young lady a few years ago who has had two kids and looks a bit like a tub you realise quite clearly and again with our pill checks we are automatically checking weight anyway and quite clearly we are able to monitor that over the years anyway. The same with antenatal work to some extent. You can see with the two or three children the weight is recorded each time so you can compare the end of the third pregnancy with what she was [when] on the pill five years ago.

Cardiac problems or potential problems through raised lipids were mentioned frequently as cues for discussing diet, as were arthritis and gastro-intestinal problems although some general practitioners identified other problems, for examples:

> If they are diabetic I suppose if they come in with a general feeling of lethargy and malaise which is [a] very common problem encountered in general practice and if there is any question [of] the child [being] hyperactive or the child being difficult they are patients that we discuss diet with quite a lot.

In summary, discussions about diet tended, not surprisingly, to originate when patients were perceived to be overweight or very overweight or when a range of specific signs or symptoms were present or when certain illnesses were being diagnosed. Certainly, there was little evidence of routine discussion about weight and diet.

Giving advice about diet-related problems

Policies for giving advice about dieting were varied. However, it was possible to distinguish between those GPs who were actively involved in giving advice and those who referred patients to a dietician, dished out diet sheets or gave pre-set diets. Obviously the two approaches are not mutually exclusive, although, as the following extract suggests, a pattern was discernible.

> I am sure that because I decided to lose weight myself my ideas have been crystallised rather in the last year. What I do now is I tell them what their ideal weight should be for their frame, size, age, and height and tell them therefore what their target weight is. If they want help with doing it and if they are prepared to work at it then we will work at it with them and again our nurse practitioner is very good at encouraging people when they become a bit low. . . . We have got a book of diets that are recommended which I think we have got ten different ones, so I tell them to get diet sheet number ten on the way out. Some of these are very specialised. We have a gastric or duodenal diet there because there are one or two patients that's relevant for and one of my partners has got a couple of faddy diets that he likes. There is a reducing diet with Edam and orange, which he enjoys and so that's one of our ten so although ten seems quite a lot I don't use more than two or three of them. Sadly our nurse prefers her own variations of the diet and so we haven't quite got our dietary policy as tight as it might be but probably the fact that they are getting a lot of advice is better than getting less.

There were, however, two approaches which were common and were related. The first of these was to 'eat much less' and the second to go on a 1,000 calorie diet. The latter advice was normally given in association with a diet sheet. Here are examples of the approaches:

> Well there I think that the principle to losing weight is to reduce your calorie intake and all the multitudinous diets which hit the market are really basically different ways of dressing up the same scheme and different approaches suit different patients. So I have no cut and dried ideas about how they do it. I can give them a simple calorie reduced diet the basis on which to work but unless they want to go on to Cambridge Diet or the F-plan diet or fruit only diet well that's fine. It's just another way of achieving the same end.

> I put most people, leaving out the pregnant, the children and diabetics, on a 1,000 calorie diet and we have leaflets which tell them about some of the food but I usually tell them to go and buy one of the booklets from Smiths but I use 1,000 calorie diets mainly.

Dieticians tended to be used if the GPs' efforts had failed although the access to and availability of dieticians were not always easy and sometimes the practices had their own 'experts'.

> Not a fixed approach but more, I would start off by checking weight myself. I would give the individual patient the opportunity to come and discuss [his or her weight] in more detail with our nurse. We don't have open access to a local dietician but we do have the opportunity to get involved with the K and C dieticians, although our nurse has been there and got a lot of practical knowledge and quite a number of different diet sheets that are kept so we would then give a diet sheet and we try and reinforce it in that way but at the end of the day the patient will decide if they come back or not.

Certainly the final comment in the last extract was reiterated by a number of general practitioners, namely, that the effectiveness of their advice depended on the motivation of the patient.

Finally one doctor said that he offered an alternative approach to using diet sheets and diet. He stated:

> I adopt a behavioural approach to losing weight. Again I am thoroughly demoralised at my efforts to get people to lose weight by using diets and diet sheets and so on. So, what I tend to do is I tend to say to them, look you know as well as I do things that you should and shouldn't eat. You can pick up any woman's magazine and you can find out from that any diet that you fancy you please yourself, you can calorie count, eat bananas, anything that you want but what I would ask you to remember is that you eat for lots or reasons, hunger being only one of them and then I go through the [other reasons, such as being] bored, the habit and the oral gratification and tension and all that sort of thing. Now I say, all I would ask you to do is before you put anything in your mouth ask yourself whether or not [you need it] or why you are eating it. If it's for hunger eat it and enjoy it and I don't care what you eat but if it's for reasons other than hunger remember that you are going to make yourself more unhappy and more overweight if you eat it. That has just as little effect as everything else and takes a bit less time and that's about it really.

Routine recording of weight and whether advice was given about diet was not prevalent. Recording of weight depended on whether it was discussed during the consultation or the person was weighed although for some diseases, such as diabetes, weight was recorded routinely. The actual recording of weight may signify to the GP that he or she has given advice about diet although there was no evidence that the actual advice was recorded or its effectiveness monitored.

Measuring serum cholesterol

The general practitioners in the sample were asked under what circumstances they took a patient's blood cholesterol. The overall picture which emerged was that serum cholesterol testing was not a common activity and was limited to specific conditions or circumstances. Three common conditions or circumstances appeared to emerge which were (a) family history; (b) if patients have signs or symptoms of CHD; or (c) if patients demand it. This extract illustrates this approach.

> The young heart attack victim. The person with a family history of hypercholesterolaemia. Often the patient volunteers it and they say, can I have a fat level done because I think someone in my family has a problem like that. If you see someone who has got obvious stigmata of too much cholesterol like the little fatty deposits round the eyes. If you get a young person who is hypertensive [this] comes as a surprise. In the older age group I am much less enthusiastic about it. The damage has been done really and it is reasonably accepted that an older heart attack victim who has a bit of a raised cholesterol is probably not worth doing much about. You might give them a token diet. The other group of people I do the test on are those who just want it done. Again, they have been reading newspapers – our practice nurses take the test and it's sent to the laboratory at Canterbury.

There were also the problems surrounding what constitutes a 'family history' and how the doctor finds out about it. One doctor suggested his work in a country practice enabled him to learn about family history because he had close contacts with different members of the family over many years. However, in many cases doctors learn through patients asking for a test because of their family history. But what constitutes a family history? The following extract illustrates some of the difficulties.

> Ask them, just say, have you got any illnesses running in your family. . . . I mean if they say their father died at the age of 56 of a heart attack then I think we would feel we were entitled [to be concerned]. . . . No, no I think it's quite an arbitrary thing. I think if the questioner is of the opinion that the individual died prematurely and I don't know how you define prematurely before the age of 70 maybe, if he died at the age of 70 of a heart attack I don't think we would but if he had a brother who had angina and a father who died of a heart attack at the age of 75 then yes we might.

A number of GPs felt that they should do it more often but couldn't because of lack of time or lack of a comprehensive screening service. Apart from the three strategies described above there were some less common ways of deciding on the need for a serum cholesterol test. For example:

> I would say probably a rough rule of thumb in the sense of looking at the person and thinking perhaps one ought to do it. I am not saying that it is entirely an intuitive thing. I think it is probably a bit of intuition and concern if you think well this is the type who might. I am not going to say to someone who is aged 50 who walks through the door, right now I think I am going to do a blood cholesterol on you . . . I would say you have got someone in fact who is in a particular age group who is a particular build, a particular weight and who is 'at risk' or you think might potentially be 'at risk'.

The actual carrying out of the test was performed either by the doctor, a practice nurse or the patient was referred to the hospital. As was shown in a previous extract, the test cannot be carried out on the spot because the patient has to fast prior to the blood being taken. Thus, it is more convenient if the practice nurse takes it or sometimes the person is sent to the hospital. For example, this was a typical response:

> Usually our practice nurse takes it. If she is not here and it's only the beginning of the day I will do it but she is here most in fact every day and so will do them. If someone comes in the evening I will usually send them up to the hospital the next day.

The actual identification of abnormal cholesterol for most doctors was not problematic because they relied on the laboratory range, for example:

> There is a normal range. I use the laboratory normal range. I don't have one in my head. . . . A lot of people feel the laboratory is too generous but then with quite a lot of people I would have a general discussion about diet, even if they are borderline, or upper normal range. I will talk about animal fats, heart disease anyway.

The treatment for 'elevated cholesterol' advocated by almost all the general practitioners was first begun with dietary advice and then maybe follow-up if necessary with drugs. However, the general feeling was that drugs were used as a last resort and dietary advice was much preferred. This was a typical response:

> Diet first for at least six months . . . low cholesterol diet, we have diet sheets. It comes down to that and they lose weight because they are usually overweight as well and then that's all if not then I'm into drugs but not for about six months.

In summary, serum cholesterol testing is not a common activity and is usually carried out when the doctors find out there is a family history, when there are signs and symptoms of CHD and when the patient demands it. A practice nurse, where available, usually carried out the test and the treatment for elevated cholesterol is usually dietary advice.

Taking exercise

When doctors asked patients about exercise their questions related to a limited number of conditions. The most common conditions were symptoms of angina and coronary related disease, for example:

> I suppose when they have some sort of heart-related condition. Well, first of all I tell them to do regular exercise rather than episodic exercise. I am sure it should be regular and I am sure it shouldn't be too severe I mean, a regular brisk walk should be the kind of level for someone with a minor heart trouble and it's really based on the kind of level.

The other conditions were obesity and muscular problems.

Certainly, there was little evidence of routine questioning about exercise and the recording of exercise in the notes was rare. Advice about exercise tended to be tailored to the health needs of the patient. For example:

> Whatever appropriate advice there is. That varies a lot, the other group of course is people who are recovering from something or a heart attack or an operation or something like that and I give different advice depending on what the situation is.

Others suggested that it should be tailored to tastes and preferences.

> I think to get them [patients] to do things that they are not interested in or do not enjoy is a total waste of time so I try and find what sort of things they would enjoy doing and are practical within their life. For example, jogging is intensely boring for most people and to advise people to jog is really a waste of breath.

However, a number of general practitioners suggested only vigorous and regular exercise was useful.

> No, obviously exercise has got to be something that doubles your heart rate so it has to be fairly energetic such as walking or go jogging or use of machines at home.

Finally, there was also the feeling that over-exertion could be dangerous, for example:

> It depends on age. If we are talking about the late middle-age group I probably wouldn't suggest jogging or doing anything too violent. I would probably suggest increased walking in the first instance.

Stress and its control

(i) Identifying stressed patients

The picture which emerged from the interviews was that stress-related problems were a major preoccupation for general practitioners as many of them discussed in some detail how they identified patients who are stressed and how they felt stress was caused. For example:

> Q. Under what circumstance do you ask about a patient's stress?
> A. I probably ask the question quite a lot in fact because it happens so often and the people who come in have got problems that, shall we say, have symptoms that are not always explained away on the basis of physical findings and I more and more these days suspect possibly that stress is underlying this so, yes, it is a question you know, what stress

are you under at work and financially or otherwise. More particularly it would be easier to ask about stress if they have got stress-related symptoms to start with when they come in.

Q. How do you identify someone who is stressed?

A. What do you mean – from the point of diagnosing it?

Q. Yes.

A. Well if someone came along with chest pains, many people come along with chest pains which are possibly or usually about angina which are caused by stress. There are many people who come along, though too many people, who have got a duodenal ulcer who are not suffering stress. That's just to quote two examples so you have got a ready-made candidate to answer the questions.

While many of the general practitioners confirmed that identifying and talking about stress was a regular occurrence, the criteria that they used to identify the stressed patient were variable. One general practitioner suggested that identifying stressed patients was relatively clearcut.

> I think that stress symptoms come in a neat little package of tired all the time, palpitations, breathlessness, maybe feeling a little bit weepy . . . those sorts of things would lead one positively to think well this person has probably got stress problems and the delight of general practice is that you know people over a long period of time and you can get a sense about when there is something physical and when there is something psychological . . . a few people come in and say, when you ask them what is wrong, 'Well, Granny has just died' and people are more and more working out those connections, but it's still novel to a lot of the population.

Not many general practitioners supported this view and some tended to suggest that many signs or symptoms were intangible and not always easy to explain on the basis of physical findings, as the first extract described. For example, the following GP suggested that they suspect stress when patients present with minor physical symptoms.

> Well either they come up and tell you that they are feeling very anxious and it is their nerves and there is all this happening and they are not sleeping, etc., or it is the patients who come with the multiplicity of small complaints and you can't really work out why they are here because nothing seems to warrant a consultation and in the end, it turns out that it is because of some form of stress in

their life such as problems in personal relationships or problems associated with work or unemployment.

Headaches were also seen as a common sign or symptom of stress and for many, stress was seen to be frequently associated (perhaps a causal influence) with heart disease. This was how one GP summed it all up.

> You get a lot a people with headaches which probably have a bearing on it. People who have high blood pressure, people who have angina, people who are anxious, people come in and cry and there are a lot of areas where stress appears to have a bearing on what is going on and I think one doesn't always say what is the problem but I think it is part and parcel of talking to people, part of the history taking, it will come to the surface sometimes, not always.

So doctors tended to look for clues and one of the commonest was posture:

> Well partly if they have got symptoms relating to coronary angina at a youngish age but mainly it's from observing them when they come in . . . there is a certain amount of body language and it's a general feeling that there is a lot of tension and stress in the situation and I think whatever their actual presenting symptoms one is then going to ask about their work.

Most doctors identified the major sources of stress as being at home or at work although as the following extract illustrates the latter source was considered to be of greater significance.

> Some of the saddest ones are people whose jobs have got [to be] a bit too much for them as they have got older and they can't really do much about it, retire early that is all. Also, people are frightened of losing their jobs and can't change their jobs now whereas they could ten or fifteen years ago. It produces a lot of unhappiness.

The difficulties of being a housewife and mother although rarely mentioned were identified by one doctor:

> I think one of the most stressful is the professional housewife who has left her profession and is battling with small children and she really feels she ought to be doing something more useful and her old man's out working, coming home telling her what a wonderful time he's had that day and there she is. I think the ones who have never been in work find it quite easy.

(ii) Managing stress

What do doctors do about managing patients with stress? The most common recipe for managing stress was what appears to be 'counselling' or talking about the problem in some depth.

> Generally I recommend that they come back and have a longer consultation with me so we can explore it further and once you have sorted out what the cause of the stress is, see how the stress can be reduced and that might mean going to a marriage guidance council or citizens advice bureau or their employer or whatever to try and sort out the underlying problems.

or:

> Q. Is it a difficult area?
> A. Extremely difficult yes because people want an answer, they want a cure this is the way I feel that they want a cure, they want me to put it right and an awful lot of the time there is nothing I can actually directly do to alter the situation at all. Sometimes it is very rewarding when one can guide them up the right alley and it works and everything is better but a lot of the time there is nothing anybody can do about the stresses and the patient is unable to deal with it themselves and it just goes on and on.
> Q. Do you use drugs?
> A. I try very hard not to use drugs. If it is a period of stress that is going to be clearly defined for a short time it's like a bereavement or an exam or a court case in the offing or something like that then I might give them you know a very clearly defined course of hypnotics or something so that they can sleep but I try not to give tranquillisers certainly.
> Q. Do patients ask for tranquillisers?
> A. Yes some do and some do not want tranquillisers but some of them are asking for something for their nerves.

or:

> I almost never prescribe drugs. I spend a fair amount of time with people. I see them again. I will try to counsel them in short bursts. I have handouts. I have a tape which I occasionally use when I have some patients in for more regular longer periods of counselling.

Other doctors were less concerned about tranquillisers as they saw that it was important to cater to individual needs. For example:

> No I don't mind [about prescribing tranquillisers] because I think one's own role is a question of treating patients. It doesn't matter to me because I am not taking the tablets; it matters to the person, but I think it is reasonable to have an open discussion with patients so that I can say, now look, I don't mind you having these, use them sensibly, if you overuse them I am going to get cross, and if you start swallowing an overdose I am going to get equally cross and I am not going to give you any more if you start swallowing overdoses. If you educate them to treat the drugs sensibly and properly, I think there is a great place at certain times for them, not all the time.

Apart from counselling, some doctors refer patients to relaxation therapists or other alternatives, for example:

> Q. What do you do about people that are stressed?
> A. I honestly suggest people go to Yoga classes or whatever and they do and it does take the top off their stress very often. They are taught to keep quiet for half an hour.

The question of whether or not to prescribe tranquillisers was obviously a dilemma for many doctors although tranquilliser use tended to be seen as a means of short-term control over the situation.

> Off the cuff two ways [of managing stress] spring to mind I guess. One is to try and say to them, well look you are not going to feel better unless the situation improves, try and improve the situation, remove the source of stress if that is possible and if it's so, well go and take a good holiday. 'I have no holiday left, doctor,' he would say. Or the other way is to say, well look if you can't get away from this stress, if your livelihood depends on it, if your livelihood depends on you rushing up and down to London working long hours you have got to do something about this and I would try and maybe give them a tranquilliser or something in fact which is not going to impair their mental faculties but allowing them to unwind a little bit. I don't really approve of giving anything that is heavy, just something to take the edge off perhaps.

In summary, general practitioners, or at least this group of general practitioners, appear to be aware that many of their patients suffer from stress-related problems and the majority stated that they tended to frequently talk to patients about how to manage these kind of issues. Also, many felt that stress-related problems were not always easy to identify although symptoms of Coronary Heart Disease were commonly believed to be stress-related. Problems at work or at home in personal relationships were seen to be the major causes of stress. Strategies for dealing with stress were, for many, problematic although the usual approach was a mixture of counselling and drugs such as tranquillisers. Many doctors were ambivalent about using tranquillisers which were generally seen as a short-term means of controlling disruptive symptoms such as sleeplessness.

CORONARY HEART DISEASE: IDENTIFICATION AND PREVENTION

Moving on from the more general views on prevention and 'lifestyle' to more specific beliefs about CHD, GPs were first asked about their views on assessing vulnerability to CHD and their views and practices about its prevention. The first few of these questions focused on assessing those who were particularly 'vulnerable'. The first one of these asked, 'How would you identify someone who is "at risk" of CHD?' For some this was not an easy question to answer as it wasn't evident that they thought in this particular way.

The vast majority, however, said that they did perceive an 'at risk' person when faced with someone who exhibited a certain cluster of characteristics, for example:

> Sometimes I mean if the classic 'at risk' person rolls in I think my goodness they really are 'at risk' you know, overweight, smoking, tense, businessmen, sort of unfit I think, oh he is heading for his MI but not in general not unless they have got really good risk factors staring you in the face.

Thus, the majority felt it was someone who exhibited the risk factors although for one the exercise was of limited value anyway:

> As general practices run at the moment there are going to be people who probably present the symptoms which [are] already too late for prevention. If you are going to prevent CHD you are going to have to start at a much younger age group and you are going to have to start with screening of the young for the acknowledged risk factors.

Concerning factors that contributed to an individual's risk of CHD many of the GPs mentioned a similar package of factors although there were some slight variations.

> Well I would say all the standard ones really, the family history, smoking and lack of exercise. Stress, it has been shown that stress is important of course it is but if it is in your personality then you are going to be affected then I wonder whether you know.

or:

> Smoking number one. Stress, prolonged stress I suppose is a number two, obesity, number three. Plus or minus high cholesterol, the bandwagon of cholesterol is slowing down really I don't think it is that important any more. High blood pressure less important for coronary artery disease than for stroke prevention, they are not sure really how much prevention of heart disease they do with high blood pressure, it is certainly helpful for strokes therefore it is worth looking for. Family history is important if your father died at forty and your grandfather did then I should think you probably could be in a bit of trouble yourself. That's the major ones.

As the quotations above illustrate, doctors had their own specific package although many of them included the same core 'standard' factors. It was noticeable that others were mentioned by some as important and not by others. There was, however, little reference to social circumstances although some did identify employment. A small group expressed uncertainty or doubt about these risk factors.

> Well yes especially the ones I have mentioned but having said that I would often make the point to people that even though they are thin and fit and unstressed and got normal blood pressure and all that sort of thing it doesn't mean that they will not be at risk of CHD because individuals are not statistics.

The third question in this group attempted to identify if there is a particular 'type' of person who is likely to get CHD. There was considerable variation in response. There are those who had a clear image as the following extract illustrates:

> I think the Type A personality, isn't it really. The active worker, the active player who plays his squash three times a week, is very aggressive with regards to his work and then drops down dead at 50.

There were others who said there wasn't a type or doubted that if there was it could explain everything or felt there was little evidence to support the Type A personality.

> There ought to be really but you can get very relaxed, lethargic people who have heart attacks and you can get the thrusting, twitchy hyped-up person who doesn't get heart attacks so I suppose there is a type but there is terrific individual variation normally.

In summary, the majority of GPs described a package of factors which put individuals 'at risk' of CHD. However, in terms of identifying an 'at risk' person or a type there was less certainty and although some characteristics were described there was a feeling that it wasn't always accurate and there was a marked individual variation.

Preventing CHD

There was only a small number of general practitioners who felt that CHD was preventable and the majority felt that they could 'minimise the onset' or 'mildly reduce' or 'modify it' or 'it can be postponed'. There were others who were even more sceptical about the possibilities of prevention. One doctor said it was due to the confusion of the evidence.

> I think that when you get so much conflicting advice like recently someone has produced a book to say that a high fat intake is of no consequence and yet for years we have been persuading people to eat less saturated fat. When you get this amount of conflict really you can't help but feel there is rather more to it than we already know. It's a bit like cot deaths in some ways that you tell mums not to overheat the kiddies and all that sort of thing and you look for the so-called 'at risk' factors, low social groups and non-breast feeding and all that sort of thing but at the end of the day you are still going to have lots of cot deaths and I suspect the same might be true of CHD that you could slim down the population, stop them all smoking, have them all eating fish and chicken and you would still have heart attacks. Maybe not as many but I still think you would have a lot.

Others thought that prevention may have a minimal effect, for example:

> I think you can minimise the onset or push off the time when you are going to get a problem but we have all got to go with something and I think anyone who dies over 75 certainly 80 should not be put

> into the statistics at all because they have got to go home with something. By the way if you ever look at statistics remember when I come to look at someone at 88 who's gone at home and one of my partners saw them four weeks ago and he seemed all right, I just look back into the register, I just look back into the thing and saw he had a stroke last time so we will give him a coronary this time or something you know are you going to do a postmortem on everybody aged 88.

These were probably the general practitioners with the more negative beliefs about prevention. The remainder, although cautious, felt prevention could be beneficial. For example:

> You can go a long way towards lessening the incident. . . . Stop them smoking. I would suggest that they have some gentle exercise as a form of both improving their cardiovascular status but of also enabling them to relax a bit. I am not a great advocate of jogging or of heavy strenuous exercise because again in my experience I have found that people can often be more stressed by having to beat a sort of time.

Finally, there were some general practitioners who were convinced of the value of prevention as the following example shows:

> In some instances undoubtedly, no doubt about that, I think if we could convince people from an early age that they should eat a sensible diet, not poison their system with too many drugs and take regular exercise, you know you're talking about educating children to do that and if they stuck to that throughout their lives then I am sure there would be a dramatic difference.

In summary, while the majority of GPs were cautious about the effects of prevention they tended to feel that prevention could have some impact particularly through controlling smoking and diet and through regular blood pressure and cholesterol checks. What of their actual involvement in CHD prevention?

Involvement in CHD prevention

For many of the doctors their involvement was what they did during the consultations, which they had described earlier in the interview. They were asked what their involvment in CHD prevention was.

> Only in the advice and the screening.

Oh nothing specifically really only just dealing professionally.

I would see anybody with CHD regularly in the surgery even if it's just to say how are you, fine off you go again. Certainly there would be other reasons for checking their blood pressure and that sort of thing but I don't screen or have any sort of programme to look for CHD.

Some weren't directly involved because clinics were available.

> Personally [I am not directly involved] but then I don't necessarily have to [be] because there are other clinics that go on.

Others, although only a small group, were more involved such as through the provision of hypertension clinics, well-man clinics and well-woman clinics. This was how one doctor described the activity of the practice.

> I think the ladies are well catered for by having a well-woman clinic which checks blood pressure and smoking history and that sort of thing. The men we have been in the process of starting up a well-man clinic and in fact we do have a practice nurse working for us, for the last year, we have actually instigated this well-man clinic one afternoon a week, one evening a week. It started off with a trial and we sent out 50 or 60 letters.
>
> Well, were they to a certain age group?

The next question focused on the involvement which the doctors would like to have in CHD prevention. The general picture which emerged showed that while the majority felt they or their practice should be more involved they were reluctant to extend their role due to lack of interest or lack of time. This was a typical example:

> Yes at least I would like to see the practice. I don't know that I would personally have the time or the inclination to do it because screening can be deadly boring. Providing you have got ancillary staff and most of this is laboratory investigations, weight, blood pressures and all these other things can be done by ancillary staff. If they count as nurses or receptionists then we get 70% reimbursement from the FPC providing our total staff does not exceed two whole-time equivalents per doctor.

Many of the general practitioners felt that carrying out the actual screening procedures was both dull and a waste of their own time, for example:

> I would like the time to persuade people who really need help to come and see me and talk about the problems that will eventually

> kill them prematurely. Not just being overweight because a lot of those will solve themselves if you solve some of the other problems which no one ever bothers about and they, I think, are probably the most important bits of it all in the job satisfaction and the unhappy relationships, domestic relationships, unhappy getting children settled. . . . This is what I personally would like to spend more time doing. The actual nitty gritty of taking blasted blood pressures all the time and weighing people all the time and so on is obviously important but I wouldn't particularly these days be too happy about spending my days just doing that . . . it is dead dull.

Time, or the lack of it, was a common reason given for barriers to more involvement.

> Obviously I would like to have [fewer] patients who have angina and heart attacks. I think the workload being as it is I don't see myself doing very much more than I am actually doing. Really one is still rushing round after the actual end result of it, the heart attacks really, strokes and so on.

Finally, there were those who were very keen to be involved.

> I think I would like to be more involved if the money was there to do cholesterols on everybody and it would be quite simple to do . . . well more so in bombarding the laboratory with large numbers of cholesterols.

Changing doctors' behaviour

General practitioners identified a number of different changes that might need to be made to encourage doctors to become more involved in CHD prevention. The most popular one of these was the introduction of financial incentives or other changes in financial arrangements for providing preventive services.

> A. Money. That is financing for the service, at the moment any form of screening that one does comes directly out of the pocket even if you get your 70% reimbursement you have still got to pay 30% out of your own pocket. Equipment [is] all paid for by the practice. OK that's deductable but [there is no] direct reimbursement over the cost of the thing. If it isn't being done on a nationwide basis, if it is being done by individuals, some form of inducement payment for the work involved doing it. If a GP is going to spend two hours a week doing a specific clinic,

then he [or she] can't do general medical work so one has to have some sort of compensation for that. I see that as the first item. The second item almost an . . . organiser if you like that's somebody who has organised one of these clinics successfully somewhere, employed either by the district or regional health authority or a colleague if you like, but somebody who can go and put their expertise into a practice and is interested and get that practice geared to doing it. GPs are often well motivated but not always terribly well organised.

Q. You did mention that coronary screening is a bit boring?

A. We are about to start a diabetic clinic here as a pilot scheme on the basis that all the items of examination will be done by non-medical personnel on the basis that doctors are pretty useless at doing routine tasks. If those tasks are delegated to other people such as nurses, etc., the routine work gets done far, far better.

Q. Is that because doctors are more interested in a wider variety?

A. I think it is partly the time factor. If you are under pressure with your clinic, looking at three or four . . . it's just another few seconds on to that consultation you tend to put it off to the next time and put it off to the next time whereas if you have got someone whose job it is to do that each time the patient comes up then it gets done.

While the majority agreed that financial incentives were crucial, some felt that if introduced they wouldn't necessarily lead to change. The previous quotation suggested organisational changes and release of more time were the key factors. Others thought that more education of general practitioners and changes in the programme of training and stronger evidence that such preventive programmes were worthwhile was needed.

I think there are quite a lot of people who say that you know it's not good, it isn't sufficient to just warn people about their smoking, tell them about their weight etc., you know people are just going to live their own sweet life as they will and is it really worth putting in all this time and effort into doing and taking all these measures and OK you pick up on or two hypertensives but . . .

The other 'change' that would need to be made now is the doctor's attitude towards prevention. One doctor referred to doctor's perceptions of their role:

It's difficult but I know a lot of doctors who don't feel that their job is to change the way that people think. There are lots of doctors who feel that their job is to deal with patients who present at the surgery and give them appropriate treatment or management and end of story . . . what you are asking is really how do you change doctors' attitudes and as a trainer I work very hard to try and change some doctors' attitudes.

Another also felt the key to the problem was the change in the approach of GPs although in a different way.

I am appalled at how many doctors do smoke . . . even those that don't smoke don't take the facts seriously enough and I am not sure whether it is apathy or whether it is lack of conviction, I think in a lot of cases it is apathy.

Finally, there was the small group which thought that prevention should be part of its role although it fitted more in the political arena.

Yes, we should be involved although the thing I feel strongest about really is that a change in our mode of living [is necessary] and that is a political matter not a medical one.

In summary, the majority felt that the key to change was through finance although this could be supported by a change in training and increase in education, more research evidence supporting prevention, change in attitude of GPs and wider political action.

Patients and prevention

The majority of the sample was uncertain if patients wanted doctors to provide these kinds of services. One group said it didn't actually know but judging by the response to cervical screening programmes it probably would. This approach is well illustrated in the following extract.

The number of women who have jumped on the bandwagon of cervical smear clinics here. The increased frequency of enquiries about a nutritionist, have you got a nutritionist, do you think if I went into the treatment room sister would give me a diet sheet, this that and the other, your cervical smears, oh yes, I think they would.

The other group was uncertain because they felt a substantial number of their patients didn't want to be involved with a doctor. This extract illustrates this approach.

I think patients don't want to be involved with doctors at all if they can help it and I think they would be much happier if prevention could be something that they acquired as a result of reading a magazine or newspaper rather than having to come down to doctors and take their clothes off. So, again we have this division of the people who most likely benefit from preventative medicine are the ones who are least likely to become involved with it and since you can never make involvement compulsory. I think that is always going to be the limited factor in any kind of scheme to reduce . . . ischaemic heart disease.

In summary the majority didn't know but felt there was increasing patient acceptance. The following quotation illustrates the general picture where some patients are enthusiastic and others sceptical.

A. I think if they are going to have some kind of screening or preventive service done they would sooner their general practitioner did it as anybody. Whether they actually want to get involved in prevention I don't know. I think it is a question of getting them to accept something as normal, a normal procedure. They have accepted having cervical smears now as normal, they have accepted having their children immunised as normal. They are beginning to accept that they can have their blood pressure checked from time to time. I don't think that there are many who are dedicated to it, there are some that are dedicated to an extreme who would go and pay £150 to have BUPA examine them all over every year or two and I am very sceptical about the value of this.

Q. You mention blood pressure screening; what about health education? Do they mind you talking about smoking?

A. Well I think the person who is smoking doesn't want to know. I think they are slightly resentful of your trying to stop them from smoking but they are the ones who one really has to talk to.

SUMMARY OF RESULTS

The aim of this chapter was to draw on evidence from a small-scale qualitative study to examine general practitioners' perspectives on CHD prevention. The majority of general practitioners in this small sample thought that, in principle, the general idea of prevention was a good one, mainly because it could help to reduce premature death.

They saw prevention as primarily involving screening and giving advice about 'risk' factors which could be carried out opportunistically or in well-person clinics. They were concerned about several aspects which were that:

(a) patients most in need did not use their services;
(b) patients' anxiety might be inflated;
(c) they were unnecessarily intervening in people's lives when they had not been invited to;
(d) they were uncertain and doubtful about the effectiveness of preventive services;
(e) it tended to create an imbalance in care and meant less emphasis on curative medicine.

These general practitioners also identified a number of problems and barriers to providing preventive services, of which the most common were:

(a) lack of time;
(b) lack of financial incentives;
(c) lack of a computerised age/sex register;
(d) low uptake of the services by patients.

Of the six activities about which the doctors were questioned blood pressure testing was the only one where attempts were made, if sometimes only haphazardly, to carry out routine screening on an opportunistic basis. Identification of smokers tended on the whole to be related to the identification of signs and symptoms associated with smoking-related disease. A similar pattern was found for alcohol use, although the identification of alcohol problems was much less common and was associated with more blatant indications such as the smell of alcohol on the breath. There was little evidence of routine weight taking, and the identification of dietary problems appears to be associated with obesity and cardiac problems. Serum cholesterol testing was not common and was confined to patients who had a family history of CHD; who had signs or symptoms of IHU; or who demanded it. The criterion on which the decision that the cholesterol level was abnormal was frequently based on the interpretation of the results by the laboratory.

The actual recording of the results of these preventive activities and the identification of problems seems to vary with the activity. Blood pressures and serum cholesterol levels were routinely recorded in the notes if and when tested. Recording of smoking seemed to be haphazard, and alcohol use and diet were rarely recorded mainly because they were rarely identified. Weight was more frequently recorded in the notes.

The actual policies for treatment and dealing with problems were, for both high blood pressure and elevated serum cholesterol, a combination of drugs and dieting. Doctors had well-defined strategies for dealing with smoking, with a range of directive and non-directive interventions on offer. Alcohol problems were more problematic; the common strategy was to refer patients with drinking problems to special clinics or centres. Dietary advice was varied, the most common approach being either to 'eat less' or to follow 'a 1,000 calorie diet'. There were considerable doubts about the effectiveness of these policies, particularly in relation to smoking.

Routine questioning about exercise appears to be rare, thus the recording of exercise in the notes was also infrequent. The policies for advising about exercise were varied and tended to be tied to the health needs or tastes and preferences of individual patients. In contrast, the identification and treatment of stress was an issue which was central to general practitioners' work, although the criteria that were used to identify 'stressed' patients were variable.

The common remedy for managing stress was 'counselling' or talking about the problem in some depth. In addition, some doctors referred patients to relaxation therapists or other alternative therapists. Many doctors used tranquillisers but were ambivalent about them and they tended to be used as a means of short-term control over disruptive symptoms such as sleeplessness.

The final cluster of questions focused on beliefs about coronary heart disease and its prevention. The majority of general practitioners in the sample identified a similar package of standard risk factors which put individuals 'at risk' of CHD. However, in terms of identifying an 'at risk' person or type there was less certainty, and although some characteristics were described, there was a feeling that these were not always accurate and there was marked individual variation.

Prevention of CHD in the main was seen as too strong a description of what general practitioners could do, the majority feeling that the most they could do was to 'minimise the onset' or 'mildly reduce' its onset. This could be achieved by controlling smoking and diet and regular blood pressure and cholesterol checks. The typical involvement (either personal or through the practice) was through case finding or opportunistic health education, sometimes supported by a well-person clinic. Although many general practitioners felt that they personally did not want to extend their role due to lack of time and/or lack of interest, they did feel the practice should be more involved, particularly in the provision of well-person clinics. There was also the general feeling that while a minority of patients were reluctant to become further involved with professional medicine, patients as a whole were increasingly accepting the value of such a service provided by their general practitioner.

With regard to general practitioners' views about what they would like to see happen in their practice in relation to CHD prevention (their personal standards), many of them felt that in general the practice should be more involved in providing mainly well-person clinics although the service should be provided, or at least partially staffed, by a practice nurse. However, in relation to specific activities there was less certainty. Blood pressure testing and smoking control were the areas where the general practitioners were most clear about what should and could be provided. Serum cholesterol testing, advising about alcohol, exercise, diet and stress were more problematic.

Finally, the key to getting general practitioners to become more involved in CHD prevention according to this group of general practitioners was the provision of stronger financial incentives and changes in financial arrangements. In addition, these doctors felt that for GPs to extend their involvement there also needed to be stronger evidence of effectiveness and changes in the doctors' attitudes to prevention in general.

This small-scale study has well illustrated the policies used by GPs and the problems that they face in the provision of services for CHD prevention. Clearly, this type of research needs to be complemented by large-scale national studies, although such evidence is not yet available. The implications of the evidence presented in this chapter are discussed along with evidence from other studies in the final chapter. However, before this we need to look at the issue from the perspective of the patient or the public.

5 Explaining patterns of health-related behaviour

One of the assumptions implicit in the proposal for general practitioners to become more involved in CHD prevention-related activities is that patients will understand and readily accept the advice given by general practitioners and will make regular use of the screening clinics. Yet, evidence from studies particularly focusing on use of medications shows that many patients ignore doctors' advice and do not take their prescribed treatment correctly (Tuckett *et al.*, 1985). However, compliance in the context of prevention may be even more difficult given that it may involve a fundamental change in behaviour. The difficulties in effecting a change in behaviour are well illustrated in the results from the field trials evaluating the impact of general practitioners' advice about smoking. The achieved changes in behaviour were quite modest never being higher than a ten per cent reduction in smoking. Also, as the evidence from Chapter 4 indicated, the problems of uptake and behaviour change are ones of which general practitioners are clearly aware.

Patient acceptance and adherence to advice appears to depend, at least in part, on the extent to which the patient is satisfied with the consultation, which in itself seems to be associated with the degree to which the doctor understands the patient's perspective and meets his or her needs. This patient-centred approach, as was shown in Chapter 3, has even more relevance for health education as the emphasis in the doctor–patient relationship is on the doctor giving advice to help patients to help themselves. In this context, the general practitioner acts as a resource in matters of health and provides skills to help the patient change behaviour.

The perspectives of the doctor and patient are in many respects different and the general aim of this chapter is to look at the so-called 'at-risk' or 'lifestyle' behaviours from the perspective of the lay person. While this portrayal of the lay perspective is of value in its own right it is of relevance to policy in that it can provide some assessment of the policy proposals and can identify the approaches that general practitioners might need to adopt if they are to be effective in health education and prevention.

The chapter examines health-related behaviour and the factors that shape it, the contexts in which behaviour changes and the barriers to behaviour change. However, the chapter begins with examining the significance of health beliefs because up until recently (Calnan, 1987), this was the traditional approach for explaining patterns of health-related behaviour.

THE SIGNIFICANCE OF HEALTH BELIEFS

This first section looks at the importance of understanding lay beliefs about health and what significance health beliefs have in explaining patterns of health-related behaviour.

There are a number of models or frameworks which have suggested that health beliefs may be useful for explaining health-related behaviour. Perhaps, the most popular of these is the health belief model. According to a recent formulation of the health belief model, (Janz and Becker, 1984) preventive health behaviour will be predicted by three sets of beliefs: perceived susceptibility (subject's perception of the risk of contracting the disorder): perceived severity (perceived seriousness of the illness/leaving it untreated – including both medical and social consequences) and perceived benefits/barriers (perceived benefits and costs of taking the recommended health actions). The idea is that these beliefs work in concert to produce a decision to carry out the behaviour or not.

An alternative construct or framework which had similar origins as the health belief model in learning theory is the health locus of control. The general principles behind the health locus of control is that people who feel they control their own health are also more likely to engage in healthy behaviour, while those who feel powerless to control their own health will be less likely to act in accordance with the recommendations of official health agencies. Since its original inception the general construct of the health locus of control has been modified (Wallston *et al.*, 1978) and the favoured approach is now the multi-dimensional health locus of control. This construct consists of three different dimensions of belief about the source of control of health: the internal, powerful other and chance. People who score high on the internal scale are more likely to believe that health is the result of their own behaviour, while high scores on the other two suggest either that health depends on the power of doctors or on chance, fate or luck.

While both these approaches have been popular there are some fundamental problems with them. These problems occur at both the conceptual and empirical levels. At the empirical level studies have shown that both models have limited explanatory power. For example, a recent study (Calnan, 1989), using data drawn from two large scale community surveys (N=4,224), examined the relationship between the multi-dimensional health locus of control (MHLC) and exercise, cigarette smoking and alcohol use. The results showed that none of these relationships was more than modest in strength even within different social and economic contexts. Obviously, this analysis does not exhaust all the behaviours. For, instance, dietary practice was not included.

Similarly, in studies examining the predictive power of the health belief model the evidence suggests only a modest relationship between the belief dimensions and behaviour (Langlie, 1979). Calnan and Rutter (1986) in their prospective study examined the predictive power of the health belief model for explaining changes in the practice of breast self-examination. Three groups of women were investigated – 278 who accepted an invitation to attend self-examination classes and were taught the techniques in detail, 262 who declined the invitation and 594 controls to whom no classes were offered – and beliefs and self-reported behaviour were measured shortly before the classes took place and again a year later. The results suggested that beliefs do predict behaviour, for both perceived susceptibility and perceived benefits/barriers made significant contributions to the belief–behaviour equations, and the relationships were generally highly reliable statistically. To that extent, the model was supported. However, the evidence also suggests that the relationship between the behaviour and the dimensions of belief which the model stresses was not a strong or a simple one. There were two pieces of evidence in particular. First, only a small proportion of the variance was explained in the analyses, which appears to be a common finding in studies using the health belief model. The figure was never higher than 25 per cent and it was generally much lower. It was also noticeable that the greatest amount of variance was explained in the control group, where the smallest amount of behaviour change was found. In fact, changes in beliefs were generally poor predictors of changes in behaviour.

The second piece of evidence was that a supplementary analysis of the data showed that prior behaviour was a stronger predictor of subsequent behaviour than were beliefs. When prior behaviour was introduced into the analysis, the proportion of variance explained was increased markedly – as far as 48 per cent in one case.

In summary, this empirical evidence suggests that the health belief dimensions identified in the health belief model and the health locus of control have limited explanatory value. In addition to the weaknesses at the empirical level there are also problems at the conceptual level.

Some of these weaknesses in relation to the health belief model have been discussed elsewhere (Calnan, 1987). One, however, which illustrates these conceptual weaknesses is an examination of the concept of perceived vulnerability. The concept of perceived vulnerability to illness in general or to a specific disease is central to the health belief model (Janz and Becker, 1984). The concept appears to be derived from epidemiological models, which, using probability theory as their basis, identify the range of factors that might influence a population's or individual's vulnerability to disease in general or to a specific disease. This concept of perceived vulnerability has been exported to the area of health behaviour where it is argued that certain levels of vulnerability are associated with a greater likelihood of compliance with officially recommended health actions. This approach has been accepted and adopted by those who are involved in designing health education campaigns where one of the major objectives is to educate the individual into awareness of how 'at risk' he or she is to certain disease.

However, when this concept was explored through an ethnographic study (Calnan and Johnson, 1985) the evidence suggested that the concept of perceived vulnerability was problematic and tended to embrace a wide range of beliefs and feelings. Respondents very rarely said with certainty that they felt vulnerable to a specific illness, although these feelings tended to be found when the respondent had some justification, such as the presence of signs and symptoms. Also, a clear distinction was made about feelings or being worried about disease such as cancer and actually thinking that they would or might get it. For some people, even thinking about the possibility of getting a disease was seen as a sign of the 'neurosis'. The possibility of getting a disease was more frequently mentioned by a respondent, although this was not based on a probability model of disease causation. The uncertainty reflected a lack of good evidence, such as previous experience of the illness in question. Certainly, the models of disease causation that predominated appeared to derive from the medical model in that the respondents tended to use criteria that characterised disease as a fundamentally biological phenomenon with a specific aetiology. Little emphasis was placed on behavioural elements, and social and economic factors were completely ignored – hereditary explanations were often used by both groups but usually as corroborating evidence in the interpretation of the significance of symptoms. According to these data, perceptions of vulnerability have little to do with health and more to do with the experience of illness and how it occurs.

A similar criticism could be applied to the health locus of control in that it focuses solely on the medical definition of health, i.e. health as the absence of illness and the extent to which there is dependence on medical professionals to manage health problems. Yet, evidence from ethnographic research has shown (Calnan, 1987) that lay conceptions of health include many dimensions such as health as being strong, health as fit and active and health as the absence of illness. Thus the instrument is probably tapping peoples' beliefs about illness rather than health and may be more valuable for explaining use of curative or preventive services, which are more concerned with the early detection of disease, or for predicting behaviour change in those with illnesses, than the 'healthy'.

Are health beliefs important for explaining patterns of health-related behaviour? This is a difficult question to answer given the lack of strong empirical evidence. Certainly, there are other dimensions of health beliefs which have been explored and might be incorporated into the model. In addition to specific beliefs, more general beliefs might be introduced, such as the value placed on health (where health is often only one of many competing values), the way health is defined, beliefs about the extent to which the individual feels responsible for his or her own health and in control of it, and beliefs about the value of disease prevention and health promotion.

Some logical connection between concepts of health and beliefs about health maintenance is evident in that a dimension of health which is very prevalent in lay concepts of health is health as being fit and active and strong. This is at least logically connected with lay ideas about health maintenance. Small-scale sociological studies (Calnan, 1987) and large scale surveys (Blaxter, 1990) have shown that diet and exercise are the most popular activities for maintaining health. For example, evidence from the National Health and Lifestyle Survey (Blaxter, 1990) showed that exercise, either in the form of active sports or keep fit, was the type of behaviour which the majority of the sample thought was the key to maintaining or improving health. Amongst the elderly, activities such as gardening were important in maintaining health where amongst the young, active sports or keep fit were important. The next most important category was diet and this was favoured more by females than males. Regular exercise is clearly logically linked with health as fitness and health as activity. The link between food and diet might also be seen as important for maintaining levels of energy and providing the resources necessary to keep active and fit to perform daily tasks.

While there appears to be some evidence of a logical connection between concepts of health and beliefs about health maintenance, how far do these concerns about health influence patterns of health-related behaviours? This particular question was the focus of a recent study (Calnan and Williams, 1991) which, using ethnographic methods, attempted to identify how salient health was in people's daily lives. The evidence from this study showed that matters of health rarely surfaced in people's descriptions of their lives and only surfaced in the context of health 'problems'; neither did a concern with health in the context of behaviour. It was only in relation to diet and food consumption that health concerns were spontaneously discussed and only by the middle-class respondents in the small sample. One interpretation of these findings is that concerns about health are not a priority for most people in the course of their daily lives nor do they arise in the context of certain lifestyle behaviours.

LAY BELIEFS ABOUT CHD: ITS CAUSATION AND PREVENTION

What of beliefs about coronary heart disease? These beliefs may influence decisions to carry out certain behaviours but they are more likely to influence how symptoms are made sense of.

Evidence from large-scale surveys and small-scale sociological studies suggests that stress is perceived by the public as being an important factor in the causation of heart disease. Twenty eight per cent of males (N=3,905) and 30 per cent of females (N=5,098) in the National Health and Lifestyle Survey (Blaxter, 1990) stated that stress and worry were important causes of heart attack. This was followed by smoking, diet and obesity. Beliefs about the causes of high blood pressure were also examined in the National Health and Lifestyle Survey. Fifty four per cent of men and 53 per cent of women said that tension, worry and stress were the major causes of high blood pressure. The next most frequent cause mentioned by both groups was obesity which accounted for 11 per cent of male respondents and 15 per cent of female respondents.

These findings were supported by a more in-depth study (Calnan, 1987) which compared the health beliefs of 30 women from professional backgrounds (social class I and II non-manual) with those of 30 women from semiskilled and unskilled backgrounds. Beliefs about the cause of a wide range of different diseases were elicited during the course of the interviews and many more of the women in the sample felt that they knew the causes of CHD better than they did other diseases such as migraine, arthritis and cancer. Of the 60 women all but 6 suggested some type of theory about the cause of CHD. These theories were usually based on a mixture of personal experience, knowledge of someone such as a relative or friend who has suffered from CHD and information they had gleaned from the media, usually the popular press. However, not many women said that they knew what a heart attack actually was like.

Many women, particularly those from a middle-class background, used multi-factorial theories of causation, as the following respondent clearly illustrates.

> Well, people have heart attacks either because they are born with a congenital heart condition which means that they are probably going to die at an early age from it or they overindulge in fatty substances, you know, for instance, eating lots or pork and fatty meats and all that sort of thing, without taking in the other things which would probably counteract the fat and I think smoking perhaps, and drinking and high living. I mean the old body can't take it all the time you've got to look after yourself. But I do think that has got a lot to do with it because is it not a fact that the arteries if you eat a lot of fat, the arteries get thicker or they get tighter and you know, restricted, therefore, the blood isn't going to the heart, therefore, the heart will find it difficult eventually but I don't know what a heart attack actually is.

Smoking and heavy drinking were specifically referred to as 'risky' activities by the middle-class women whereas lack of exercise was exclusively referred to by the working-class women. The importance of hereditary factors was also identified by both social classes although they were perceived as having a lesser role in the cause of CHD compared with other illnesses such as cancer, arthritis and migraine.

The other factor that was frequently identified by the middle-class women was the effect of stress and strain. Obesity and stress and strain were also the conditions that were the most popular with the working-class women although these women placed relatively more importance on the risks associated with stress and strain. Particular emphasis was placed on the stress and strain from overwork:

> I mean men work today up to such a point. I mean because things are so dear I mean they have got to work up to such a point to keep up with the living, haven't they? Women today go out to work a bit more that is why they have bad hearts and all this sort of thing because they are doing their housework and then rushing back again. I think in this country today we are in a rat race to keep going. I think it's just fast living.

The extent to which individuals were perceived to have control over the onset of heart disease or have responsibility for the onset of heart disease was explored in a later study (Calnan and Williams, 1991). Certainly, there was little evidence of personal responsibility or blame about the onset of heart disease and respondents did not agree with the view that those who suffer a heart attack deserve it or that their illness is a punishment which they have brought upon themselves. For example these were typical accounts:

> That's a load of nonsense. Heart attacks, some people have defective hearts, some people cause their hearts to be defective by smoking, I suppose you could say they deserve it in a way, but in the case of a smoker it's self-induced, obviously the person who has been born with a defective heart can do very little about it.

> Rubbish. A heart attack, people can bring heart attacks on themselves by overwork, stress, worry a multitude of reasons, or it can be just a natural way of the body telling you to slow down or there may just be a malfunction in your heart and no matter how fit you are, just something suddenly goes.

Certainly, compared with other diseases, such as AIDS, there was much less moralising about heart disease. For example, this was a typical response about whether individuals who contract AIDS deserve it.

> Well, if you are daft enough to use a dirty needle and stick it in your arm, you get what you are asking for. If you are sleeping around with the wrong people or indeed anybody, and you know you don't have the right precautions, you're asking for what you get. That's a very broad view, but there's always the unlucky one who gets, you know, smitten by whatever just because his number's up. I'm a great believer in fate.

IMAGES OF THE PERSON LIKELY TO GET CHD

Lay people's beliefs about disease causation have been shown not only to contain ideas about the causes of disease but also often contain stereotypes about the types of people likely to get a disease (Cowie, 1976). With some diseases, such as cancer, no pronounced stereotype was found. Anybody was seen to be 'vulnerable' and, as one women stated 'it is no respecter of colour or creed'.

However, with CHD a clear stereotype was evident. The type of person most likely to develop CHD was described by women from both the middle and working-classes as the anxious and nervous type. For example, this was how one respondent described the type:

> I think people who are hyperactive who don't really know how to relax.

The respondents' theories about cause, not surprisingly, influenced their images. Thus, those who were overweight, or who overindulged or who were under stress were seen to be particularly at risk. The relationship between stress and work was identified by both social class groups but its meaning seemed to vary. For example, this was how one middle-class woman described the relationship and, as will be seen, there was an indication of a perceived difference between the risks associated with gender:

> Well, I suppose it's the classic case of the business-man who eats and drinks too much, it seems to be a fairly common theory doesn't it? And I think stress has a lot to do with it. I mean I have known of people who have had to make a lot of their staff redundant and soon after they've finished work, they've had a heart attack, so obviously if you are a worrier that can happen.

In contrast, the working-class women placed less emphasis on the mental pressure of stress and more on the physical elements:

> I always put it down to him working on building sites for some reason. I don't know why . . . too much lifting, carrying.

THE PREVENTION OF CHD

Nineteen of the 30 women from professional backgrounds stated that CHD might be preventable, although only two appeared confident that it could be prevented. The belief amongst this group was that prevention was of value because it might 'reduce the possibility' or 'lessen the risk' of getting the disease. While only nine of the 30 working-class women said that heart disease was preventable, the majority of these (six) felt that it *could* be prevented.

The middle-class women who thought that heart disease might be prevented emphasised the value of not smoking, moderate drinking, eating a careful diet and having regular exercise. This was a typical response:

> I think you can reduce your chances of having heart disease by not smoking, not overdrinking and not getting too fat.

Regular exercise and diet were also activities referred to by the small group of working-class women who thought heart disease was preventable. However, the importance of controlling stress and strain through taking life easier or slowing down was also highlighted by this group as the following extract shows:

> I think you can [control stress] by taking the pace of life slower because to me a lot of people rush and if they slow down a bit then I think it would be a lot better.

This identification of the importance of stress and strain in the causation of heart attacks appeared to be one of the major reasons why many working-class women were doubtful about the preventability of heart attacks. They felt, as the following quotation illustrates, that they had little control over the source of stress and strain:

> I don't think [I have much control over stress]. I think only try to avoid stress and worry and I think in today's society you have got stress and worry anyway. So I don't know.

Exercise and the prevention of heart attacks

The idea of preventing heart disease through adopting certain life-styles was further explored by examining respondents' ideas about the relationship between having regular, physical exercise and the prevention of heart disease. Women were asked specifically if they felt activities such as jogging would help prevent heart disease.

The middle-class women tended to be uncertain or doubtful about its value. A minority (three) thought it might be valuable because it was relaxing or because it 'strengthened the heart'. The remainder were more doubtful about its value and although many saw the positive qualities they tended to weigh them against the costs such as the dangers of bringing on a heart attack. The working-class respondents were even more sceptical about the value of jogging and the small group who did see its benefits described them only in terms of keeping fit. However, many working-class respondents were strongly against it as the following respondent illustrates:

> Well, I think all that sort of thing is silly, I think jogging can give you a heart attack quicker than anything.

Evidence from other studies of lay beliefs about disease causation has shown how lay beliefs often parallel scientific theories in terms of structure and content, even though as a system of beliefs they may lack the same level of coherence. Lay beliefs about CHD causation are no exception in that emphasis was placed on stress and strain and diet and weight. Also, a clear image of a 'type' of person who was likely to get CHD was portrayed which, in some respects, paralleled the Type A personality.

An understanding of lay beliefs about disease causation is important, not least because it might indicate how far people feel they can control or influence the development of a disease (Pill and Stott, 1982). In some diseases, such as cancer, biological or hereditary factors are perceived by lay people as being the most significant causal factors which are believed to be outside the person's control. In the case of CHD, however, it was shown that behaviour and environmental circumstances were important. It is difficult to judge how far people felt they could influence these causal factors. The middle-class women, in particular, felt that changing lifestyle factors such as diet and smoking might prevent CHD and implied that this behaviour was, to some extent, within their control. However, the working-class women appeared to be more doubtful about the preventability of CHD, particularly as the major causes of it, stress and strain, were generated by the way society was currently organised which was perceived as being outside their influence.

In summary, while there is some evidence that health beliefs have a significant influence on patterns of health-related behaviour the traditional instruments for measuring health beliefs only have a limited explanatory value. For example, the health locus of control was only modestly associated with health-related behaviours. One possible direction may be to examine the relations between beliefs about control over other, perhaps more important, aspects of an individual's life, and health-related behaviour. For example, activities at, or associated with, work may shape a large proportion of the population's perception of the world. Thus, it might be useful to examine the relationship between beliefs about control over work and health-related behaviour.

Cornwell (1984) in her ethnographic study amongst working-class people in London showed how living and working conditions shaped not only beliefs about health but also beliefs about other aspects of social life. She found that the set of moral/philosophical assumptions which underlay beliefs about work were similar to those which underlay beliefs about work. Differences or inequalities in occupational status and income were believed to reflect the natural order of things and most people do the work that naturally suits them which is itself influenced by natural abilities such as level of intelligence. Thus, it was felt that people had little control over the job that they did, although they did have some control or responsibility for how they went about their work. Similar dual theories were prevalent in her subjects' accounts about health and illness. While 'being healthy' depended on whether or not one was naturally endowed with a good 'constitution', good health also had to be earned through leading a life of moderation, virtue and hard work. In this respect, people had little control over their health because it depended on differences in constitution but they could control or have 'responsibility for' their health by having the right attitude.

A more detailed investigation of the relationship between the work environment, beliefs about control and health-related behaviour might begin by focusing on the process or the way that the restructuring of the work environment actually influences beliefs about control. For example, Karasek (1979) distinguishes between two elements of the work environment at the individual level which are the job demands placed on the worker and the strategies adopted by the worker to cope with these demands. Thus, the extent to which the individual feels job strain and control over his or her work will be influenced by the degree to which the conditions of work enable the management of job demands. This in turn shapes beliefs about control over other aspects of life such as health and will influence beliefs about health-related behaviours.

What do patients want?

Another fundamental assumption in the policy proposal emphasising the role of the general practitioner in prevention is that patients should want their general practitioners to be involved in prevention, particularly in health education. A number of surveys have suggested that the majority of patients do wish their general practitioners to be involved (Fowler, 1986) in prevention. Although, as Wallace *et al.* (1987) show, patients are rather selective about what they want their GPs to do. For example, when the patients were asked whether their general practitioner should be interested in their lifestyle the proportion who gave a positive response, in both sexes, was highest for weight and lowest for drinking. Also, more patients recalled having received advice about weight than about any of the other aspects of lifestyle, and few had been given advice about drinking. Other consumer surveys (Williams and Calnan, 1991) have suggested that the lack of advice given by GPs about lifestyle was a major source of patient dissatisfaction. Reasons given by patients (Calnan, 1987) for doctors' lack of involvement in this area were the doctors' attitudes, because patients only consult when they are sick or as the following respondent stated, doctors suffer from 'a lack of time' for dealing with prevention.

> Well yes, but the doctors never have enough time, do they? Um, you know, to think about how to keep people healthy. They are so engrossed in how to cure people when they are ill.

However, perhaps more interestingly, the idea of health promotion held by the respondents was shaped by respondents' concepts of health. For example, some respondents defined health as the absence of serious illness and this advice about health maintenance was seen in terms of advice about illness, as the following extract illustrates:

> I think they should advise you more than they do. Obviously, if you go with the same complaint time and time again he should look into that more to find the root of the trouble as to why it keeps recurring and not just giving you the same tablets to take time over and over again because that's not curing the root of the problem.

EXPLAINING PATTERNS OF HEALTH-RELATED BEHAVIOUR

The first part of the chapter focused on health beliefs and their possible association with health-related behaviour. The conclusion that emerged was that certain dimensions of health beliefs are important but their explanatory power is not strong. The aim in this next section is to examine alternative explanations for patterns of health-related behaviour.

Evidence from empirical research has shown that the strength of the statistical interrelationships between types of health-related behaviours are at best modest. For example, in one study (Calnan, 1989) using a random sample from a community population (N=4, 224) it was found that correlation between alcohol use and smokers

(0.19) and alcohol use and exercisers (0.15) was positive but only modest in strength. A similar pattern emerged in a large National Health and Lifestyle Survey (Blaxter, 1990) which examined the interrelationship between smoking, alcohol use, diet and exercise. This study examined the interrelationships between behaviours in different age and gender groups. The highest correlations were between smoking and diet with those who smoke being more likely to have a poor diet, and those who do not smoke a better one. Smoking and alcohol were also associated but less strongly and alcohol consumption was associated with a high level of exercise. For men, drinking was correlated with a poor diet but diet was not correlated with exercise. However, for women, a good diet was correlated both with a high level of exercise and a low level of drinking. But, once again, the strength overall of the correlations was never more than modest (<.25). The implication of this is that health-related behaviour cannot be conceptualised as a uni-dimensional phenomenon.

Evidence from a wide variety of sources (Townsend *et al.*, 1988; Blaxter, 1990) has also shown that patterns of health-related behaviour vary markedly by socio-demographic characteristics such as social class, age, gender and educational background. Not only that, but clusters of behaviours tend to be found amongst certain social groups. For example, Blaxter (1990) shows that those who were smokers, drinkers, had a poor diet and carried out a low level of exercise were more likely to be men, to be unskilled manual workers, to be unemployed among the young and living alone among the elderly. Twice the average rate of this pattern of behaviour was found in the Northern and Yorks/Humber regions. However, as Blaxter (1990) clearly shows, this type of group was in the minority and the majority did not have totally healthy or unhealthy lifestyles.

One interpretation of these pieces of evidence is that while individual beliefs about health-related behaviours or beliefs about the consequences of the behaviour may influence the decision to adopt the behaviour in question, social and economic circumstances may provide a setting which can act to enable or constrain the practice of health-related behaviour.

Beliefs and behaviour

In the previous section the importance of health beliefs were discussed. However, there are other social psychological models which focus on the health-related behaviour itself and beliefs about it. For example, there is Fishbein and Ajzen's (1975) theory of reasoned action. According to this model, behaviour which is under conscious control is predicted by 'private' beliefs about the consequences of performing the behaviour and 'normative' beliefs about the behaviour which are the perceptions we have of how others believe we should behave. In other words, the theory of reasoned action already includes the most powerful predictor from the health belief model – the perceived value of the behaviour, but adds normative beliefs to the equation. Empirical evidence (Calnan and Rutter, 1986) on mothers' choice of infant-feeding methods, women's decision to use cervical screening and breast self-examination demonstrates that normative beliefs play a highly significant part in behaviour and that normative beliefs and 'private' beliefs together predict behavioural intentions more successfully than do 'private' beliefs alone. A similar approach has been used by Sutton (1987, 1989) in his research on smoking which had focused on decision making and consideration of the perceived consequences of the available courses of action. For example, people might perceive that the benefits of smoking in terms of stress reduction tend to outweigh the costs which might include the health risks.

This approach is well illustrated in the study by Marsh and Matheson (1983) in their national survey of 2,700 smokers. This study examined the possible link between smoker's attitudes, intentions and behaviour. They specifically wanted to explain why one in five of those smoking ten years ago no longer did so. The researchers suggest that the traditional view of psychology of smoking, that the habit is controlled by nicotine dependence, may be useful for explaining why people continue to smoke or why ex-smokers frequently return to the habit. However, it contributes nothing to why there are so many people giving up.

Marsh and Matheson (1983) investigated the influence of attitudes on changes in smoking behaviour. According to their data the development of positive attitudes towards not smoking led smokers to try to give up. These attitudes take one of three basic forms. Those who try to give up seem to develop a belief in the general benefits of not smoking (money, social gains and so on). They also develop specific beliefs about the positive health benefits of not smoking. Finally, they may also develop the belief that giving up smoking no longer poses the threat to their mental equilibrium that they once may have feared. This leads the authors to conclude that smoking is a psychological dependence that, in most smokers, is learnt under the special emotional conditions of adolescence. It may just as easily be unlearnt by a process of attitude change.

Others, using a qualitative methodology, have attempted to identify the circumstances or context in which behaviour change occurs. For example, Saunders and Allsop (1983) show that many problem drinkers give up drinking of their own accord once the drinking begins to pose a problem for them as distinct from being a problem for other people. For example, the formation of a new social relationship, a change of job, moving house or the development of a health problem may bring the drinking sharply into focus in a context which is meaningful and important.

Hunt and Mcleod (1987) carried out an exploratory study using qualitative methods to examine what makes people change their behaviour. They found that there was little evidence that changes in health-related behaviour were a response to formal health messages. Most changes followed a long period of thought, often of an intermittent nature and these tended to be sporadic attempts at change before a successful outcome was achieved. Reasons given for behaviour change were varied although health was in a minority. These included financial for smoking and diet, change of social scene for smoking, diet, exercise, drinking, family problems for tranquillisers, vanity and problems with clothes for diet and self-esteem for tranquillisers.

Data from this study also highlighted the interrelationship between different behaviours. For example, one respondent who was very active in sports said that she did it in order to off-set her smoking and alcohol intake. The connection between losing weight, maintaining weight and smoking was a very strong one especially for women: 'smoking helps to keep my weight stable'. 'I'd rather smoke and keep the weight off. I couldn't handle being fat again.' Also, there was an interrelationship between the use of different addictive substances: 'I drink a lot. I prefer it to pills' or 'If I stopped smoking I'd go on drugs'.

From their data the authors concluded that:

> For most people health-related behaviours exist, normally, at a mature level: for example, smoking, the amount of exercise taken, the kind of food bought and eaten, having a drink, are largely built into the flow of every day activities in a way which is not vulnerable to 'health messages' since these behaviours are integrated into the social relationships and adaptive processes which are part of the meaning system of an individual's life.

Social position and health-related behaviour

Evidence, as has been previously stated, also shows that patterns of health-related behaviour vary markedly by social position and it is therefore necessary to concentrate on the structural factors which modify beliefs, and circumstantial factors which enable or constrain intended or preferred courses of action.

Social and economic factors may act in a variety of ways. For example, studies, such as that of Cornwell (1984), have shown how people's general beliefs about health and the extent to which they feel they have control over their daily activities are shaped by their position in the social structure. Blaxter and Paterson (1983) have shown how 'low' norms about health are adopted by those living in circumstances of social or economic disadvantage due to the relatively greater experience of ill-health suffered by this group.

Calnan's study (S. Calnan, 1989) focused on the way old people view health, illness and disability and how this relates to the way they view old age. The data were obtained from interviews with a sample of 96 people aged 75 or over. There was evidence of a negative stereotype of old age in general held by old people themselves which was closely linked to ill-health and particularly disability. However, the respondents tended to be 'optimistic' about their own health despite suffering a certain amount of disability. They used illness and disability as evidence that they were old, and people who felt they were old were likely to see their ageing as a consequence of ill-health.

Calnan (S. Calnan, 1989) also found amongst her sample of old people evidence of a duality of beliefs about the control of illness in old age and of old age itself. People felt both that it was possible to maintain their health as they got older and also that their health was bound to deteriorate as they got older. However, when it came to their own experience they seemed to opt either for the fatalistic view of illness and old age as irresistible or the optimistic view of both illness and old age as resistible through will-power. Those who took the former view tended to be the ones who saw themselves as old and those who took the latter tended to be the ones who did not. Thus, whether people see themselves as old is of significance if a prediction is being made about the likelihood of their seeking out and co-operating with health care services for their ailments.

Alternatively, there is an approach that places greater emphasis on the direct impact of the circumstances in which people live and work. This approach is well illustrated in the work of Graham (1989) who showed how the interrelationship between socio-economic circumstances and gender influenced the individual's attitude to smoking. Graham (1989) shows that at both household and individual levels, the evidence points to substantial spending on tobacco by low-income households. For example, low-income households with two adults and two children devote an average of 5 per cent of the weekly household income to tobacco, compared with 2 per cent in all households with two adults and two children. In addition, they spend absolutely more on tobacco than other households. Also, spending among low-income households with children is higher than among those without children. The highest expenditure on tobacco, calculated on a per capita basis, is among one-adult households with children; 90 per cent of these are headed by women. Studies have also shown (Baldwin, 1985) that there are higher levels of spending on tobacco among households with a disabled child at all income levels. Thus as Graham points out:

> The research indicates that spending on tobacco is strongly related to particular forms on inequality, and specifically with caring for children in poverty.

Graham (1989) through her qualitative investigation, also provides an explanation for this pattern. In her study of 57 women she showed how in some families smoking was associated with breaks from care, when they rested and refuelled. She showed that cigarettes were also associated with breaks in their pattern of care when the demands of the children were too much to cope with. As one woman stated (Graham, 1989):

> Sometimes I put him outside the house, shut the door and put the radio on full blast, and I've sat down and had a cigarette, calmed down and fetched him in again.

In the context where women had to cut back on any luxury goods for themselves such as shoes, haircuts, etc., cigarettes could be a woman's only purchase for herself. Thus, smoking reflects the social isolation and stress of caring for children in poverty. As Graham concludes:

> Where smoking is part of an individual's response to disadvantage, it is likely to function as part of a complex array of coping strategies that maintain the fragile equilibrium of every-day life. In these circumstances, increasing the pressures on women to become non-smokers may have wider implications for individual and family well-being. These may be missed by people concerned only with smoking cessation.

This is a good example of the relationship between social structure and individual health-related behaviour. Another area where there is a relationship between social position and health-related behaviour is in patterns of food consumption.

Food consumption involves the consumer in a range of interrelated activities which include food purchase, food preparation and cooking, and the serving and consumption of meals. Each of these activities is influenced by a variety of factors associated with wider socio-economic circumstances and with the internal structure of the family, such as gender roles, the division of labour in households.

The most extensive research into the social organisation of food consumption in households was carried out by Charles and Kerr (1986a, b, c, 1987) in 1982 and 1983 on a sample of 200 women with pre-school children, living in a Northern town and its surrounding villages. This study combined a detailed exploration of attitudes with the use of a diary to document actual practice in the households. They found that women were, in the main, responsible for buying, preparing and cooking food within families. This responsibility, however, does not necessarily mean that they determined and controlled what they and their families ate. Indeed, they tended to subordinate their own needs and preferences to those of other family members, particularly their partners and to a lesser extent their children's preferences. Men's involvement in tasks such as food preparation was minimal and the amount of 'help' they gave to their partners depended on their availability and goodwill. Cooking was also regarded as an integral part of a woman's role as wife and mother, and many women tailored what they cooked to fit or to please their partners. Charles and Kerr (1987) also found that foods were ranked hierarchically in terms of social status and their distribution in the family reflected the relative power and status of a family member. Thus, adults tended to consume high and medium status food such as meat, fish, eggs and cheese and children tended to consume low status food such as biscuits and baked beans.

Men's foods appear to be higher status than women's food, which reflects lack of status. Women tended to share food with the children and therefore women's food consumption occupies an intermediate position between that of men and children. A similar pattern was found by Graham (1987) in her study of lone mothers and food choice. She shows that lone mothers no longer had to adapt to the food preferences of their male partners, cooking meals their men liked. When they had partners, the women's food preferences were 'eclipsed and reshaped to conform to the choice of their partner. . . . Thus, she showed that as with money, there is a tendency to separate the control and management of the family diet'. The lone mothers still catered for children's preferences but also had greater freedom as they gained control and management, which meant they could improve their diet according to their preferences and economised more effectively.

While these data clearly illustrate the relationship between gender and patterns of food consumption what of the relationship between social and economic position and food consumption and health? There is clear evidence of differences in consumption patterns between different income groups. The National Food Survey (Central Statistical Office, 1989) showed that in 1986 people from low income groups were eating more processed meat products, whole milk, eggs, lard, sugar and jam, cakes and biscuits, and canned and dehydrated soups than their more affluent counterparts. They were also eating more bread and potatoes, and most of that bread was white bread. At the same time, they were using less low fat milk, cheese, canned meat, poultry, fish, green and root vegetables, fruit and wholemeal and brown bread.

What of the explanations for these different patterns? One explanation suggests that there are differences in health beliefs between different social class groups because of the uneven impact of health education. However, there is little evidence to support this. For example, in one study (Calnan, 1990) where women were asked for their perceptions of good and bad foods, healthy and unhealthy foods, and balanced and unbalanced diets, the results indicated that both groups had a good understanding of current nutritional messages. In Wales, the percentage of people believing that 'being overweight' and eating foods high in animal fat are an important contribution to the development of disease varies little between social classes (Heartbeat Wales, 1987). Certainly there is considerable evidence that many people from disadvantaged backgrounds are unhappy with their diet and are not eating the diet that they would choose.

Calnan and Cant (1990) asked directly what the major influences were on food choice as perceived by the main purchaser of food in middle-class and working-class households (see Table 5.1). In both sets of social classes the predominant influence was family likes and dislikes. The second most common influence was concerns about health suggesting that both groups were equally concerned about health although the middle class appeared to be driven more by health knowledge than specific health problems.

Explanations for the link between social class and patterns of food consumption have suggested that internal factors within the household may be the problem. For example, some have argued that the pattern of influence within the family may also vary according to the particular sub-culture to which that family belongs. Thus the less educated and lower-paid husbands often exert more influence over decisions in their family. Other explanations have emphasised that it is the inequality in resources available in the family that limits the influence of working-class women. Pill and Parry (1989) found in their study of 130 working-class families, that attempts made by the women to initiate changes for themselves or for the family as a whole may be thwarted through lack of support from husbands and, to a lesser extent, children. The data from group interviews suggest that this is at least partly due to a lack of resources since women, the people normally responsible for household tasks, have neither the time nor money to cater for a range of dietary requests from different family members.

This was one of the conclusions arrived at by Wilson (1989) in her

Table 5.1 Influences on food choice as perceived by main purchaser of food

Influences on food choice	*Social classes I & II*	*Social classes IV & V*
Family likes and dislikes	10	11
Needs (pragmatic)	2	-
Attitudes and expectations	1	-
Health: problems	2	4
knowledge	9	5
Diets and slimming	2	4
Quality	3	-
Cost	2	3
No influence	1	-

Source: Calnan and Cant (1990)

study of 61 families living in an inner city area of North London. She examined the barriers to dietary change both within the household and outside. She found that while there were gender differences in food preferences and tastes in the family and that women were responsible for food purchase and preparation, most women could change their family diets if they wanted. However, there were some exceptions and these were those people on low incomes. She argues that there is little evidence for the so-called cultural or class-based constraints on dietary change. The major restraints arise out of low incomes and the household financial arrangements that disadvantage women. Thus, she found that only in families with low incomes or where the family budget left little for food was finance a barrier to dietary change. The amount of money available for collective domestic consumption was vital because in the poorest household there was no question of the mother meeting her own preferences. Thus, the pattern of food consumption in households was determined by financial arrangements inside and outside the family.

Certainly, as Cole-Hamilton (1989) pointed out, many of those from households living on low incomes did not eat their preferred diet. However, within the constraints of their budget Cole-Hamilton, drawing on data from the National Food Survey, showed that people with low incomes buy food considerably more efficiently than those with high incomes. They received more for their money, both in terms of quality and also in nutritional terms. Both in 1983 and 1986 people with low incomes were buying nearly every type of food more cheaply than the national average price. The proportions of the household food budget spent on different types of food also show that people with low incomes are more likely to spend a larger proportion of their scarce resources on the types of food which are recommended in a healthy diet.

What of the cost of a healthy diet in line with current dietary advice? Cole-Hamilton argues (1989):

> All the evidence collected over the last 4 years points to the fact that the cost of a diet in line with current dietary advice, which takes into account individual preferences and social factors, costs significantly more than the amount most people with low incomes in the UK are able to spend on food.

This is well illustrated in Table 5.2 which shows the percentage price increases between 1982 and 1986 for foods which were encouraged in a healthy diet and not encouraged in a healthy diet. The figures appear to indicate that the price increases in healthy 'foods' were far greater than those for 'unhealthy' foods (see Cole-Hamilton 1989).

In addition to cost there are other factors which influence food choice. One of these is availability: Cole-Hamilton (1989) shows that recommended foods for a healthy diet were less likely to be available in deprived areas than in more affluent areas. Costs of an individual's diet not only include the costs of food but also the expenses incurred in buying food e.g. transport costs to and from shops. Local shops or the mobile shops tend to be used not because of quality but because of convenience. The costs of time and money (many do not have cars) outweigh the benefits of shopping in a supermarket where the food may be a better quality and cheaper.

The studies described so far concentrated on smoking and diet only. A more recent study by Calnan and Williams (1991), while also looking at health-related behaviour in a social context, examined the relationship between social class position, gender and smoking, alcohol use, dietary practice and exercise. Using material gathered from in-depth interviews with middle-aged couples (both partners were interviewed) from social classes I and II (professional) and IV and V semi-skilled and unskilled, the general aim was to discover why certain social class settings encourage and others discourage the adoption of certain patterns of health-related behaviour. This study adopted a novel methodology at least in this area of research. The interview focused on a day in the life of the respondents. The interviewer's brief was to try to elicit a detailed chronicle of the day's activity and specifically to identify the salience of health beliefs and the respondents' perception of health-related matters.

Some of the more interesting and illuminating results from this study were found in the analysis of the data about exercise and fitness. Certainly, this analysis revealed fairly striking differences and points of divergence between social class groups regarding both health beliefs and health-related behaviour located within the context of the respondents' daily lives. The first point of divergence between the social classes concerned the issues of the subjective perception of, and satisfaction with, their general level of 'fitness'. Thus, a generally inverse relationship between social class and satisfaction with their current level of 'physical fitness' was found. That is to say, those in social classes IV and V (semi-skilled and unskilled) generally seemed to be more subjectively satisfied with their current levels of fitness than their more affluent counterparts who, instead, were generally more likely to express a sense of dissatisfaction and a desire to be 'fitter' or to improve their current level of fitness still further. These respondents often cited being over-weight, even if only slightly, or not taking enough exercise as reasons for this.

Table 5.2 Changes in prices of 'healthy' and 'unhealthy' foods

Foods encouraged in a healthy diet	*1982 p/1b*	*1986 p/lb*	*% increase*
Cereal foods			
Wholemeal bread	26.65	31.19	17
Brown bread	26.86	32.54	21
Breakfast cereals	55.56	70.59	27
Potatoes	7.18	7.88	10
Fresh vegetables			
Cabbages	17.01	19.97	17
Cauliflower	19.79	23.58	19
Other green vegetables	43.07	64.99	51
Salad vegetables			
Leafy green	41.49	55.47	34
Cucumbers	35.42	48.66	37
Tomatoes	40.23	52.04	29
Roots & other vegetables			
Carrots	14.76	17.93	22
Onions etc.	17.55	23.79	36
Miscellaneous	37.36	52.99	42
Fresh Fruit			
Oranges	23.88	30.42	27
Other citrus fruit	26.03	35.96	38
Apples	28.82	33.55	16
Bananas	30.17	43.72	45
Fruit juice	20.02	32.89	64
Poultry	69.18	86.88	26
Herrings	66.74	85.86	29
White fish	107.26	154.05	44
Yoghurt	52.91	69.46	31
Vegetable & salad oils	38.41	46.05	20
Foods not generally encouraged in a healthy diet			
Cereal foods			
White bread*	20.08	23.05	15
Other breads*	42.75	50.23	18
Buns, cakes & pastries	71.24	90.74	27
Biscuits	76.87	91.31	19
Sugar	19.84	22.43	13
Beef & veal+	147.42	164.87	12
Mutton & lamb+	113.13	128.48	14
Pork+	102.86	122.19	9
Bacon & ham	115.99	131.02	13
Sausages	70.23	80.04	14
Whole milk*	20.12	23.61	17
Butter	83.52	91.44	9

* White bread and whole milk play an important role in many people's diets, but wholemeal bread and reduced fat milks are generally encouraged in current nutrition education

\+ Carcass meat is not discouraged per se, but people are generally advised to eat leaner, more expensive cuts, and to cut down on fatty cuts.

Source: Cole-Hamilton (1989)

The second striking difference with respect to social class, concerned both the nature and the definition of what exactly 'physical fitness' and 'exercise' constituted and involved. While most respondents appeared to accept that exercise had a beneficial effect on health status, those in social classes IV and V (semi-skilled and unskilled) tended to have a far more pragmatic or functional definition of physical fitness, one which was grounded in their ability to perform or function in their normal daily activities. 'Exercise' was far more closely tied in people's minds to the tasks, activities and duties involved in carrying out vocational and domestic roles. For example:

> Q. Would you describe yourself as physically fit?
> A. Oh yes.
> Q. In what way do you think you are fit?
> A. Well . . . I have got quite a physical job and I do not get [any] aches and pains, I feel quite healthy. I get the odd colds, but I feel quite healthy . . . I do not think I could be fitter than I am now. I'm quite fit anyway.

In contrast, whilst an ability to function in one's normal daily roles and/or an absence of disease/illness was also referred to by those in social classes I and II (professional), they were far more likely to stress 'fitness' in terms of 'athleticism', strength, stamina and so on; being fit in a far more technical sense over and above one's ability to perform one's everyday activities. Partly as a consequence of this, and partly due to the nature of the work engaged in (i.e. non-manual) their conception of 'exercise' tended to transcend normal daily roles to encompass things like swimming, squash, badminton, golf, cricket, keep fit and aerobics classes, use of gym, horse riding, climbing and skiing. Furthermore, in addition to the widespread recognition, referred to earlier, of the health-promoting effects of exercise, there was also a tendency amongst this social class group to stress and emphasise the diffuse sense of 'well being' which it generated and the contrast and the relief which exercise provided from daily activity and obligations. The following comment was fairly typical of the middle-class group's perspective.

Q. Would you describe yourself as physically fit?
A. Not just at the moment I wouldn't.
Q. So why do you think you are unfit?
A. Because I have always been quite involved in sport and over the last year I haven't played so much sport and I haven't had so much exercise, I have got a bit lazy and I wouldn't call myself fit at the moment.
Q. So would you like to be fitter than you are now?
A. Definitely yes.
Q. In what way?
A. Well, I get a few aches and pains and I think if I wanted to play sport now I would find it, certain sports like squash, I would find hard work, because I have got out of the habit and that did keep me fit and hockey to a lesser extent.
Q. Do you carry out any activity to keep fit?
A. Not regularly, I did go to a gym, but then we got busy and I didn't go, and I haven't been back.

The study (Calnan and Williams, 1991) also examined alcohol use within the context of the respondents' daily lives. A number of interesting findings emerged. First, it was clear that individuals tended to operate with quite different notions of what exactly terms such as 'moderate drinking' actually mean. Moreover, although the pattern was far from clear cut, it seemed that those in the middle class, deemed to be drinking 'a lot', tended to be regarded by those within the working class, who consumed a broadly similar amount per week, as only 'moderate' drinkers. Secondly, the data demonstrated the degree to which both alcohol and drinking are woven into the very fabric of contemporary social life, forming a part of what it is to be sociable.

Many respondents, irrespective of social class background, spoke of how drinking tended to occur, particularly within the home, only in the presence of guests and visitors or on special occasions such as Christmas, birthdays, wedding anniversaries, 'high days' etc.

> Well, we buy lager for Christmas and we always have a bottle of white wine in the cupboards. We would probably drink lager for Christmas and probably, if we had visitors, friends come, then we will open a bottle of wine. That's about the extent of it.

However, there were interesting social class differences. Whilst examples could be found of working-class respondents who only tended to drink at home, if at all, and of middle-class respondents who tended to drink in pubs etc. the more frequent pattern was for working-class drinking to centre around pubs and clubs – especially at the weekends – as *an end in itself*.

> A. Weekends we go out, Friday, Saturday and Sunday.
> Q. And where do you go then?
> A. Usually just round the club, the Working Men's Club or the local pub.

In contrast, the middle-class respondents displayed a somewhat different orientation; one in which drinking was either more home-centred, particularly with friends or *with a meal*, or alternatively tied to vocational and recreational roles duties and obligations, hence being more an accompaniment to some other end. The following accounts were fairly typical with the second reflecting the tendency not to frequent the pub.

> We do but not a lot, more for social occasions rather than everyday or anything like that. . . . When we have visitors, when we have people for a meal, that sort of thing, and then we would bring a bottle of wine out . . . Last Thursday evening we had visitors, I think I had a Cinzano and lemonade and two glasses of wine. . . . Some weeks none, just if we have visitors, which I suppose we have about every other week.

> Not really no, I don't frequent public houses, it just doesn't appeal to me, the social atmosphere.

Thirdly, there were clear gender divisions in relation to drinking with men tending to rate themselves as heavier consumers of alcohol than women and, as the following quotations testify, this gender difference was perceived as something only to be expected:

> I mean I don't drink as much as my husband, because I think men do don't they, you know.

> I think men have this chauvinistic idea that they must not be seen not to have a drink and they often tend to drink more than they want and it can make them ill.

Fourthly, and finally, alcohol use was the only behaviour where beliefs were ambivalent about the link with health. All respondents appeared to accept the fact that the consumption of alcohol, when taken to 'extremes' or consumed 'excessively', could cause harmful effects to health. In short, the dangers of alcohol for health were both well recognised and, publicly at least, appeared to be well heeded. However, respondents displayed a generally ambivalent attitude towards alcohol and alcohol consumption. Indeed, the ideas of drinking in 'moderation' being a pleasant, sociable, relaxing pastime – some even stressing its beneficial, health-promoting effects – together with the darker side of 'excessive' alcohol consumption, were dominant themes within many of the respondents' accounts. The following quotation illustrates the positive, sociable, relaxing side of drinking.

> Oh it's relaxing you meet people, passes a couple of hours away.

The notion of 'moderation' was also expressed.

> Q. Do you think drinking is good for people?
> A. It doesn't do them any harm in moderation.
> Q. Why do you think that?
> A. Well anything in moderation is good for you.

Then there was the *negative*, darker side of drinking, for the drinker.

> Oh yes it can cause all sorts of problems, I mean a mate of mine, I used to go round there before we was married when we lived in Essex and he could get paid on the Thursday and be skint by the Friday.

A somewhat different aspect of how alcohol may bring out the 'darker side' of one's personality is expressed below.

> I have never found it harmful. . . . No, I think what I don't like is the violence it generates in some people. I think it is probably hidden in there in their character anyway and the drink problem enhances what is their normal character.

This study, along with the research on smoking and food consumption, highlights the necessity of placing health-related behaviour in its broader social context. It is only then that the whole logic of people's action in relation to other aspects of daily life can be grasped, assessed and appreciated.

In summary, this section has focused on the factors that influence health-related behaviour. The early part of the chapter suggested that examining beliefs about the behaviour or the meaning placed on health-related behaviour might be a more useful approach to understanding behaviour than focusing solely on beliefs about health, or the health-related aspects of behaviour. The latter parts of the chapter indicate how important it is to see health-related behaviour and the meaning placed on it within its socio-economic context. The examples of smoking, alcohol and patterns of food consumption clearly illustrate how the social circumstances in which people live and work shape their 'style of life'.

Attitudes or social circumstances?

Explanations for variations in patterns of health-related behaviour, as was shown in the previous section, either tend to emphasise the importance of individual attitudes towards behaviour and its consequences or the importance of the social context and circumstances in which the behaviours are carried out. The evidence suggested that both explanations were significant and were probably interrelated. However, Blaxter (1990) in her analysis of data from the National Health and Lifestyle Survey, attempts to estimate the relative effects of circumstances and attitudes upon behaviour. In her study she found that health beliefs, such as a general, positive orientation towards responsibility for health, or, internal locus of control, or measured in terms of beliefs about the importance of specific behavioural factors for health were associated with behaviour. People with positive attitudes or beliefs that behaviour is important were more likely to adopt 'healthy' lifestyles. The aim of this analysis was to find out to what extent the connection between attitudes and behaviour is due to intervening characteristics such as income, education, family, social class or region of residence.

Some of the evidence which emerged from the analysis suggested that attitudes have rather little effect upon behaviour if social circumstances were controlled. For example, in her causal analysis examining differences between 'healthy' and 'unhealthy' behaviour she examined the relative importance of attitudes such as the internal locus of control against social class and income. The causal analysis shows that, within social classes and income groups, locus of control has a negligible effect on behaviour. The total effect of social class is partly through income and partly through education.

In summary, it appears that health beliefs may be of little importance for explaining patterns of health-related behaviour. The evidence suggests that other dimensions of belief such as beliefs about the behaviour itself may be of greater significance. Increasing evidence also points to the importance of social structural factors such as social class, age, gender and education. Some studies have begun to identify the possible explanation for the link between social position and smoking and this research has been extended into other areas such as exercise and alcohol use (Calnan and Williams, 1991).

The implications of this evidence for general practitioners appear to be that giving patients advice about the health risks of certain patterns of behaviour may be useful in raising patients' awareness and possibly will lead to a change in beliefs. However, if the aim is for general practitioners to be more 'interventionist' and attempt to change behaviour then the task is more complicated. As the evidence suggests, it may be more useful for general practitioners to focus on the beliefs about the behaviour itself and attempt to grasp what the behaviour means to the individual. However, a strategy of attempting to change individual behaviour may not be sufficiently effective given that many health-related behaviours are closely tied to social contexts and social circumstances. General practitioners would therefore need to pursue policies which are aimed at social change as well as at individual change. Some of these policy options have already been outlined in Chapter 3. These approaches would concentrate on breaking down the barriers and constraints within the wider social milieus which impede changes in health-related behaviour.

6 A conclusion

The aim of this book has been to consider the prospects and policies for the prevention of Coronary Heart Disease and the political and social circumstances which have shaped the development of policy in this area. In this final chapter, the intention is, in the light of the evidence and the arguments presented in previous chapters, to discuss the issues and the implications for future policy.

GENERAL PRACTITIONERS AND PREVENTION: A POLICY FOR INDIVIDUAL OR SOCIAL CHANGE?

The policy analysis in the previous chapters suggested that exhortations for general practitioners and the primary health care team to become more involved in prevention came from a number of different quarters. Doubts about the efficacy of modern, hospital-based scientific medicine along with the need to develop a distinct professional identity were some of the reasons, why, over the last decade the official representatives of general practice pursued a policy advocating a shift from 'curative' to 'anticipatory' care. This policy has, at least over the last five years, been supported by another powerful actor, i.e. the government. In the White Paper on primary care and in the new contract great emphasis has been placed on increasing general practitioners' and the primary health care teams' involvement in health promotion. While this may be a result of pressure by the profession or other interest groups there are other reasons for the government's increasing involvement in this area. One of these reasons appears to be economic in that prevention is seen as an inexpensive option as it may lead to a reduction in demand for expensive, technological medicine. Another reason is ideological in that the White Paper's discussions of prevention would seem to reflect the state's current predilection for encouraging individual responsibility and self-care.

The two most influential actors in the development of the policy exhorting general practitioners to become more involved in prevention have been the medical profession itself and the government. However, two other actors also played a part although perhaps to a lesser degree. One of these is the pharmaceutical industry. The pharmaceutical industry has always had a close involvement with general practitioners and seems to be one of the major sources of information for general practitioners. Certainly, in the area of prevention of coronary heart disease it has been argued that the pharmaceutical industry is actively encouraging cholesterol testing to increase the prescription of cholesterol lowering drugs (Vines, 1989). For example, in a recent survey, Sharp and Rayner (1990) found that of primary health care team members who carry out cholesterol testing 15 per cent were using desk top machines to measure cholesterol concentrations in blood samples and the remainder were using local hospital laboratories. The use of a desk top machine seemed to increase the number of cholesterol tests done and the majority who used these desk top machines were loaned them by the pharmaceutical industry. Sharp and Rayner (1990) conclude:

> The least expensive desk-top machine costs more than £4,000 – a non-reimbursable expense which must inhibit their widespread use in general practice. On the other hand the loan or gift of a machine by a pharmaceutical industry has been encouraging cholesterol testing in primary care. We believe that this practice may fail to conform with the ABPI code of practice for the pharmaceutical industry.

The pharmaceutical industry, therefore, appears to have a vested interest in the increased involvement of the primary health care team screening for risk factors for coronary heart disease. The fourth actor, who also has taken a lesser role up until now, is the patient. As evidence in Chapter 5 showed, the majority of patients wanted their general practitioners to be involved in preventive activities although it is difficult accurately to assess the influence of the patient on policy developments. The general practice setting, because of its structural characteristics, is vulnerable to the influence of the patient, although the evidence suggests, at both the individual and collective levels, patients have had little impact on the development of general practice (Calnan and Gabe, 1991). This may change, however, as disposable incomes rise, at least amongst some groups, and consumers are and will demand a wider range of choice and will want higher standards of service. Higher standard of service will involve preventive care and currently much of this is being provided by the private sector. However, for many people this is seen as an expensive and unpopular option and there will be increasing pressure from consumers, or some groups of consumers, for general practitioners to expand the range of services available, particularly into fields such as preventive medicine.

In summary, there are a range of actors who have encouraged general practitioners to have an increased involvement in prevention. While the representatives of the profession initiated the policy other actors, such as the government, the pharmaceutical industry and the patients have more recently encouraged this development.

The analysis also raised a number of important problems about the general practitioner's role in prevention. Some supporters of the policy (Calnan and Johnson, 1983) argue that general practice is the natural setting for prevention not least because they have frequent contact with patients and because their registered list of patients permits a systematic approach to local population screening and audited follow-up, with unique access to manual-worker groups which are at higher risk of diseases such as coronary heart disease. In addition, supporters of this approach have referred to evidence of the success of packages of health education interventions used by general practitioners aimed at controlling cigarette smoking. Also, there is some crude evidence that GPs' advice about smoking-control is a cost-effective method of reducing CHD.

While the analysis showed that there was considerable support for increasing the involvement of the practice teams in prevention it also raised a number of critical issues. Perhaps one of the most critical issues was whether the general practitioner was the most appropriate person to carry out such a role. Certainly, the assumption appears to be that given effective communication by doctors and nurses and well resourced and organised screening and recall systems then most of the patients' problems can be resolved. Some have suggested that this policy is a good example of medicalisation in that the medical profession, or some sections of it, are deliberately trying to expand their jurisdiction into areas of social behaviour. However, from the evidence presented in Chapter 4, such an argument is simplistic in that the majority of the general practitioners were hesitant about being involved in advising about alcohol, food consumption and to a lesser extent smoking. Many of them felt that they had not been trained to deal with these problems and were sceptical about the effectiveness of their interventions.

The problem, as was clearly shown in Chapter 5, is that many of the behaviours have social origins and thus it may be more appropriate to effect change through public health and social policy rather than to attempt to effect change at the individual level. Thus, doctors are being asked to practice prevention and health promotion when the causes of illness are not within their domain. However, this is not to say that general practitioners cannot or do not have a role to play in social change. As was shown in Chapter 3, there are at least two 'collectivist' roles they can play. One has a more paternalistic, public health orientation where the general practitioner acts as political advocate. This is very similar to the role that the BMA has been playing in the recent deliberations on the White Paper and in the smoking debate. The other is a more community-oriented role where the professionals and the public work together. However, there are potential pitfalls and problems in simply exhorting GPs to get involved in community education programmes. To begin with, while the public may accept the GPs advisory role during consultation and in the surgery, it may not as readily accept that role within the community at large. Self-help groups, community action groups or community health projects may be more acceptable and effective in this context. Furthermore, community involvement would require a major paradigm shift for general practitioners: one-to-one consultations and contact with patients and their families is the modus operandi and main daily experience of GPs. In addition, many of the shortcomings and biases identified in the 'prevention in general practice' debates are common to medicine as a whole. The present system of selecting and training doctors, and their prevailing medical subculture, both can prevent significant changes from taking place.

One alternative or perhaps complementary policy option to general practice is to make the workplace the setting for the provision of preventive programmes. Certainly, it might increase the likelihood of participation by 'at risk' groups such as men and people from unskilled and semi-skilled occupations. However, there are disadvantages not least of which is the lack of any national occupational health service. Also, the employer may see such a scheme as a form of capital investment aimed at increasing productivity by maintaining a healthy work force and may shape the programmes with this end in mind. In addition, for the employee there is the question of confidentiality in that employers' knowledge of employees' health status may jeopardize their employment and career prospects.

There are, however, stronger arguments for developing a more coherent national policy at a number of different levels than for focusing solely on the primary health care team. A combination of regulations, fiscal policies and education strategies can provide the necessary environment for effective interventions by the primary health care team. One area on which policy discussions have recently focused is the development of a coherent smoking control strategy. The evidence has suggested that a package of measures, including large increases in the price of cigarettes, health education campaigns and legislative control over tobacco advertising, could be a very effective method of reducing cigarette consumption. However, as was pointed out in Chapter 2, it is important to assess the social and economic costs of policy options. Thus, policy makers have to come to terms with the realities of the economics of tobacco and policies need to be developed which cope with these economic changes, such as the fact that the tobacco industry is a declining industry in affluent countries.

Policy makers also need to take into account the social implications of their strategy. A health policy for smoking which uses a number of measures, including a pricing policy and education, may only create guilt and anxiety in groups whose circumstances are such that they would be unable to change their behaviour if they so wished. This was well illustrated in Chapter 5 which presented evidence about how women bringing up children and living in poverty were unable to change their smoking habits even if they wanted to. In addition, as Cameron and Jones (1985) point out, our society not only needs alcohol, tobacco and other drugs of solace to relieve individuals of a great burden of pain and suffering but could not function in its present form without them. Also, as Crawford (1984) showed in his study of concepts of health amongst middle-class Americans, there are two apparently contradictory definitions of health which are prevalent. On the one hand, to be healthy is to demonstrate that there is concern for the virtues of self-control, self-discipline, self-denial and will-power. On the other hand, health means being happy, enjoying oneself and being free to indulge oneself as one wishes. Thus, it appears in Western society there is ambivalence about the use of drugs. However, for those with adequate resources – time, energy and finance – it may be possible to change to the use of a less harmful drug or engage in activities which compensate for the effects of the drugs. However, for those without such resources the costs of the change may outweigh the benefits.

Similar issues are relevant to the equally important but less developed area of food and health policy. While a range of policy options have been mapped out in this area, the evidence to evaluate the most beneficial course of action to follow is not yet available (see Chapter 2). For example, Winkler (1987) offers an imaginative outline of the possible options for food health policy in relation to CHD prevention. He identifies a number of different strategies which could be carried out in combination or independently. First there is the education strategy. Winkler (1987) (see also Sanderson and Winkler, 1990) states that most of Britain's present effort of raising nutritional standards is educational in character, but grossly under-funded and directed solely at consumers. He suggests that other groups such as doctors, food scientists, agronomists, caterers, food marketers etc. should be targets for education and there should be an improvement in the nutritional component in the training of these occupations. He suggests also the introduction of a comprehensive system of nutritional labelling for all manufactured foods. The second strategy, the substitution strategy, uses other commodities in place of harmful ones. As Winkler points out, Britain's agriculture, food manufacturing and retailing industries are constantly innovative in the products they produce and processes which they use. At present, little of the change is directed towards nutritional improvement. Winkler recommends a programme which positively adopts nutritional principles; such could include (a) altering the composition of manufactured foods to reduce the salt and fat content, (b) reallocating health budgets away from curative towards preventive medicine, e.g. away from heart transplant operations to nutrition education campaigns and (c) instituting a research and development programme to produce palatable substitutes for salt.

The third strategy is a pricing strategy, which encourages switching from harmful to healthy commodities by altering their relative prices. He argues that many government financial policies already affect patterns of food consumption but they are instituted for economic reasons without taking nutritional considerations into account. This strategy involves lowering the prices of healthy foods and raising the prices of harmful foods. Examples of specific policies might include (i) the reorganisation of the agricultural price support system to stop encouraging the production of fatty milk, (ii) differential rates of VAT related to the nutritional value of the foods, (iii) the cessation of discounted supplies of EEC surplus butter to food manufacturers and government caterers and (iv) the restoration of excise taxes on salt, similar to the present taxes on tobacco, alcohol and petrol, which are also designed to control consumption.

The fourth strategy, the provision strategy, would directly affect consumption by improving the food provided in government institutions. The government is the nation's largest caterer. Meals are provided in schools, hospitals, crèches, day centres, old people's and children's homes, military bases, prisons, in the canteens of government offices and nationalised industry plants and via meals on wheels. The potential for improvement is great and might include a range of specific policies such as the introduction of national criteria for school meals and the extension of them to all other forms of government catering services, nutritionally-orientated specifications for all manufactured foods purchased by government and the regular monitoring of nutritional standards of food provided by government institutions.

The fifth and final strategy is the regulation strategy. Current food law guards against dangerous additives, unhygienic processes and inferior ingredients, but does little to raise nutritional quality. Much other law (e.g. on taxes or imports) affects food consumption without being recognised as 'food' law. Winkler (1987) recommends a number of improvements which include transfer of the responsibility for food regulations from the MAFF to the Department of Health, the alteration of grading systems for carcass meats to encourage the production of leaner animals and the replacement of existing compositional regulations for manufactured foods with new nutritionally-oriented standards.

Clearly, then, Winkler (1987) outlines a range of policy options for government and other agencies in the area of food and health which specifically relates to heart disease. The policy options are not exhaustive but illustrative of the various alternatives available. The next stage is to collect evidence that can lead to a rigorous evaluation of the possible impact of the different policy options. It might be that, as was shown with smoking control, a 'package' of measures is the most effective strategy.

This approach would place the general practitioner and the primary health care team within the context of a coherent policy pitched at different levels. However, it does not mean that the GP should be divorced from local health policies at both a planning and developmental level. As the empirical research shows, general practitioners have few links with and limited knowledge of health education and preventive activity beyond the practice. One way of encouraging this approach would be to attach a 'facilitator' to general practices. The facilitator could help GPs and other members of the primary health care team to develop links with the community, particularly with health education units as well as voluntary groups.

GOVERNMENT POLICY AND HEALTH PROMOTION IN GENERAL PRACTICE

Policy documents prepared by the official representatives of general practitioners (see Chapter 3) have at least three different arenas in which GPs could be active in preventive activities. One of these is the consultation, another is the practice population as a whole and the third is the local community. However, as the empirical research (limited though it is) has shown, there is a marked discrepancy between the rhetoric of the policy proposals and the reality of preventive practice in the consultation and at the level of practice.

Evidence from the local studies suggests that general practitioners are interested in prevention and health education and believe that the general idea of prevention is a good one mainly because it could help to reduce premature death. Prevention was perceived as primarily involving screening and advice-giving about 'risk factors' which could be carried our opportunistically or in well-person clinics. However, there appears to be marked variation in doctors' actual involvement and in their policies for risk assessment. For example, blood pressure testing performed mainly on an opportunistic basis was the most common activity and identification of smokers appeared to be increasingly common. Routine questioning about alcohol problems, routine weight taking and identification of dietary problems and routine questioning about exercise were less common. However, stress or stress-related conditions were common problems presented to general practitioners and for many this was seen as part of their risk assessment policies.

There were also marked variations in treatment policies or policies for dealing with 'problems' in behaviour. Elevated blood pressure and smoking appeared to pose little difficulty for general practitioners although they found alcohol problems difficult to handle and the majority were referred to specialist centres. Dietary problems and elevated blood cholesterol also proved to be problematic and many general practitioners appeared to have difficulty in interpreting the epidemiological evidence about which patients to treat. Drugs, sometimes in combination with health education, were the commonest form of treatment for elevated cholesterol. However, policies for reducing obesity were variable. Stress and stress-related conditions were usually dealt with through counselling or through drug treatment. Many general practitioners saw the latter approach to be useful in the short term but the use of tranquillisers was not seen as a long-term solution.

What of the explanations for the marked variation in involvement? The published evidence which examines the barriers and obstacles to involvement relies heavily on general practitioners' self-report and perceptions. Some of these explanations pinpoint the importance of the doctor who has more interest in curative medicine, is confused about the epidemiological case for dietary change or is sceptical about the benefits of prevention and his or her ability to change behaviour or finds prevention and health education 'dull and boring'. Alternatively, others suggest the problem lies with patients in that they do not wish their GPs to provide preventive services or do not use the services when they are provided. A third type of explanation suggests that the problems lie outside of the control of doctors and patients but are inherent in the current structure and organisation of general practice. Poor facilities, lack of purpose-built premises, lack of computerised age/sex registers, lack of support staff are all common explanations for variation in involvement. Also, a lack of time due to a heavy workload because of the demand-led nature of general practice is an explanation frequently put forward.

It is difficult, given the lack of available evidence, to identify which if any of these is the most powerful of the barriers. The evidence from the qualitative study suggests that general practitioners do suffer from both a lack of knowledge about policies for intervention and a lack of support from suitably trained staff for their initiatives. Certainly, the lack of clear evidence about the relative importance of risk factors is confusing both to general practitioner and patient. Not having access to a reliable source of information about these issues has led general practitioners to rely, perhaps too heavily, on the pharmaceutical industry for information.

The lack of time due to a heavy workload is a common explanation used by general practitioners (also taken on by their patients) for not being able to be involved in prevention. Yet, in a study examining the relationship between doctors' list size and their involvement in prevention (Butler and Calnan, 1987) no significant association was found. Similarly, no significant relationship was found between involvement in preventive activities and hours spent in practice and non-practice based activities (Calnan, 1988a). One implication of this evidence is that even in circumstances which enable general practitioners to have more time to expand their services into new areas such as prevention there still will be a marked variation in provision. This variation may be explored by focusing on demand-led factors such as the social composition of the patient load and by supply side factors such as the practice style of the doctor and the level of support received from other members of the primary health care team. However, as the study described in Chapter 4 clearly showed, from the GP's point of view the key to getting general practitioners more involved in CHD prevention is through the introduction of stronger financial incentives and changes in financial arrangements.

This policy has, in some respects, been taken up in the government White Paper on primary care and has been implemented in the new contract. These proposed changes in financial arrangements aim to increase the reliance of a doctor's income on capitation and fee for service payment. It is an attempt to improve the range and quality of services available by making doctors pay 'more performance' related. Thus, the emphasis on capitation is intended to reward the 'competitive' GP who increases or maintains market share as indicated by patient list size.

What impact will this proposal change in financial arrangement have on the supply of services provided by general practitioners? Will it lead to an increased provision of services aimed at CHD prevention? Under the new contract a fee will be paid for checking the height, weight, blood pressure and urine of newly-registered patients over five years old. In addition, all patients between the ages of 16 and 74 who have not consulted a doctor within the past three years will be invited for a check up. While doubts have been expressed about the take-up rate of the non-consulters and the benefits of urine testing for the presence of glucose, overall this should increase the number of patients receiving health education and screening. However, the new contract and the 1987 White Paper have tended to adopt a restricted view of prevention in that emphasis is put on a 'medical model' of screening. Moreover, detection of 'at-risk' patients as well as the necessity to produce quantifiable results means spending time on medically – rather than socially-oriented problems. Also, it has been argued that under the new contract consultation lengths may decline rather than increase. For example as Morrell (1989) points out:

> Overall, the contract is imbued with the belief that 'good care', as it defines it, will attract more patients to the doctors providing this care, and the doctors will consequently receive greater financial rewards through a system of payment based largely on capitation. It ignores perhaps the most crucial aspect of primary care, which is concerned with the time doctors can devote to listening to and identifying their patients' problems and to providing counselling, advice, health education, and appropriate management.

This argument appears to be partly supported by the evidence (Calnan and Butler, 1988) that as list sizes increase the number of hours worked in the practice and outside the practice increases but the length of consultation decreases. Hence, the time available, particularly to carry out health education in the consultation, may diminish along with the quality of care.

Similarly, the payment of a sessional fee for clinics aimed at CHD prevention or preventive activity may well lead to an increase in the number of clinics provided at the expense of quality. For example, as Forbes (1988) points out when commenting on the experience of fee for service systems in Western Europe, 'The popularity of fee for service, however, has been tempered by the side effects of this payment system. The most frequent criticism is that doctors have a clear incentive to increase the quantity of the service irrespective of any improvement in the service quality'. Also, as Robinson (1989) points out, health screening and health promotion aimed at the affluent worried well might become more attractive to general practitioners because of their revenue earning potential at the expense of less money-spinning services such as long-term care for the chronic sick. This criticism applies both to the new contract and 1989 White Paper with its proposals for general practitioners to become budget holders. In addition, there is the possibility of a shift in the balance of preventive care away from routine opportunistic screening in the consultation towards clinic-based preventive activities where the financial rewards are more lucrative.

Others (Horder *et al.*, 1986) are even more sceptical about the value of financial incentives for changing GPs' behaviour and they conclude: 'The evidence on the effects of existing financial incentives is mixed; these incentives seem to have encouraged more activity in some areas but not in others.'

In summary, the evidence suggests that the shift in the system of professional reimbursement for general practitioners away from a mix of capitation and salary (allowance) towards a greater weighting for capitation may lead to an increase in the provision of a range of preventive services but might also lead to a reduction in quality. However, there are other aspects of the new contract which might encourage more involvement. One of these is the incentives towards computerisation. At present, estimates suggest only one in eight practitioners regularly use computers in consultation rooms yet the presence of a computer is crucial for any effective screening programme and for follow-up. Also, activities such as blood pressure testing should be facilitated by the abolition of restrictions on the range and numbers of staff that may attract reimbursement. Thus, general practitioners may in future be able to employ the greater numbers of staff and the greater variety of staff, for instance dieticians, that a properly supported programme will require. Similarly, in the new 'budget practices' greater incentives will be needed to employ practice nurses and other ancillary staff to handle much of the routine procedures at lower cost. While such a policy may be economically sound there are still some doubts about whether staff are adequately trained in prevention to carry out such tasks.

The major question seems to be whether the practice nurse will perform an instrumental role acting as a complement, probably a subordinate, to the general practitioner or if he or she will act as a substitute to the doctor becoming fully involved in health education and counselling. From the patient's point of view, nurses may be more accessible than doctors although little is known about the nature of the relationship between practice nurse and patient and whether it is conducive to effective health education. Early evidence from field trials (Coronary Prevention Group, 1990) shows that smoking cessation advice by nurses is not very effective, at least, compared with advice given by general practitioners. Recent evidence (Coronary Prevention Group, 1990) also shows that primary health care teams involved in health examinations have a very limited understanding of nutritional principles and doubts have been raised, therefore, about the value of dietary education from these sources.

Finally, there is another implication of the recent government proposals for changes in the health service (DHSS, 1989) and for the provision of activities aimed at CHD prevention in general practice which needs to be considered. It was suggested in Chapter 3 that health education was a crucial part of CHD prevention yet the current social organisation of the doctor/nurse/patient relationship tended to be a major obstacle to effective education. For example, Tuckett *et al.* (1985) in their study of how general practitioners and patients communicated, showed the majority of consultations were one-sided; doctors did little to encourage patients to present their views and there was little discussion of the consequences of a patient's illness. However, as was suggested in Chapter 3, for general practitioners and nurses to become more effective educators they needed to adopt a more patient-centred approach, to show greater versatility and flexibility in their professional role and to move away from a specialist towards a more general role. The doctor and nurse would adopt the role of the counsellor giving the patient the reassuring advice and support 'for them to help themselves'. The emphasis would be on the general practitioner to shift towards the practice of a more holistic or socially-oriented type of medicine. Will the recent government proposals encourage such a shift?

The answer to this, at least according to some commentators, is no. For example, as Bartholomew (1989) states:

> The emphasis on quantifiable behaviour in the White Paper proposals could shift general practitioners from the practice of holistic or socially oriented medicine, towards more medically oriented behaviour . . . while health promotions and preventions are given importance in 'Promoting better health', these are only measurable as screening and immunization targets and health checks . . . while prevention and health promotion and are an accepted part of general practice care, they will now involve considerable resources being diverted into audit requiring sophisticated information systems. The added requirement for practitioners to now negotiate within the internal market for hospital services, is to shift the emphasis from the doctor as independent professional to that of bureaucratic functionary.

One implication of the new proposals is that general practitioners will increasingly move to a more managerial and bureaucratic role with their interests being determined more by financial than professional concerns. Certainly, general practitioners are being put in the position of mediator between the financial concerns of the government and the more professional concerns of patient care. This appears to be antithetical to the development of a more patient-centred approach.

Yet in the government proposals there appear to be conflicting policy aims. On the one hand there is emphasis on financial accounting and value for money while on the other emphasis is placed on the need to be more sensitive to patient demands. Certainly, in these policy documents there is considerable rhetoric about 'consumer sovereignty' and the 'enterprising consumer' although specific recommendations are made in the areas of demand which are aimed at creating a structure which leads to greater consumer choice and control. How effective such a strategy will be is difficult to judge. Some argue (Haigh-Smith and Armstrong, 1989) that the proposals show little understanding of what consumers want from general practice and are based on:

> normative criteria of good quality originating from both medical and government sources. Criteria valued by the consumer varies according to age and sex, and the best way of maintaining patients' satisfaction seems to be to emphasize the traditional if

> more intangible virtues of good general practice encapsulated in the attentive, competent and available doctor.

Thus, while doctors may be required to become concerned with meeting consumers' demands the actual relationship between them and their patients may become more formal and bureaucratic and consequently may neglect the specific wishes of the patient.

In conclusion, the proposals in the new contract and the White Paper on the Health Service should increase the likelihood of the general practitioner and the primary health care team providing services which are more likely to be tailored to some consumer demands, such as increased provision of preventive services. Also, the emphasis on the introduction of a comprehensive system of audit should improve the standards of service available in general practice. However, these changes may have two kinds of costs. On the one level they may lead to a deterioration of the doctor–patient relationship and on the other, they may bring about the provision of unnecessary services, the creation of an imbalance in care and the development of further inequalities in the provision of services. General practitioners may find themselves as mediators between the government's requirements to control spending and the consumer's requirements to maintain or increase standards of care which includes the provision of preventive services. At present, many consumers turn to privately-funded health care for preventive medicine. However, with increasing costs and rising premiums for private health insurance, consumers will increase their demands for an expansion of the range of services available in general practice under the NHS and in particular they will wish to see expansion into fields such as preventive medicine. Thus, the general practitioner will have to come to terms with the conflicting roles of business manager and professional although recent evidence (Corney and Calnan, 1991) suggests that the increased managerial and administrative role is not one that most general practitioners particularly enjoy. Much will depend on the role and involvement of other members of the primary health care team, particularly the community nurse, and the level of support given to general practices by the Family Health Services Authorities. The latter have a particularly crucial role although their influence may depend to a large extent on the priority they place on health promotion, their perception of their role in terms of whether they take an active or passive stance in relation to the development and implementation of policy and the nature of their managerial relationship with general practitioners.

References

Aaron, H. and Schwartz, W. (1984). *The painful prescription: rationing health care*. Washington: Brookings Institute.

Armstrong, D. (1979). The emancipation of biographical medicine. *Social Science and Medicine*, 13A, 1–8.

Atkinson, A. and Skegg, J. (1974). Control of smoking and price of cigarettes – a comment. *British Journal of Preventive Medicine*, 28, 45–8.

Atkinson, T. and Townsend, J. (1977). Economic aspects of reduced smoking. *Lancet*, ii, 492–4.

Baggott, R. (1986). Alcohol, politics and social policy. *Journal of Social Policy*, 15, 4, 467–80.

Baldwin, S. (1985). *The costs of caring: families with disabled children*. London: Routledge.

Balint, M. and Norell, S. (1975). *Six minutes for the patient: interactions in general practice consultation*. London: Tavistock.

Bartholomew, J.E. (1989). Working for patients in general practice. Unpublished MSc dissertation, Royal Holloway and Bedford College, University of London.

Bartley, M. (1985). Coronary heart disease and the public health. *Sociology of Health and Illness*, 7, 3, 289–313.

Beaglehole, R. (1986). Medical management and the decline in mortality from CHD. *British Medical Journal*, 101, 825–36.

Beattie, A. (1991). Knowledge and control in health promotion, in Gabe, J., Calnan, M. and Bury, M. (eds) *The sociology of the Health Service*. London: Routledge.

Berkmann, L.F. and Seeman, T. (1986). The influence of social relationships on ageing and the development of cardiovascular disease. London: *Coronary Prevention Group*, 175–82.

Bjartvert, K. (1977). The Norwegian Tobacco Act. *Health Education Journal*, 36, 3–10.

Bjartvert, K. (1986). Smoking control policy in Norway. Paper given at Social Medicine Society meeting, London.

Blaxter, M. (1990). *Health and lifestyles*. London: Routledge.

Blaxter, M. and Paterson, A.S. (1983). *Mother and daughter: a three generational study of health, illness and behaviour*. London: Heinemann Educational.

Bond, S. (1950). BMA report on preventive care. London.

Borhani, N.O. (1985). Prevention of coronary heart disease in practice: implications of the results of recent clinical trials. *JAMA*, 254, 2, 257.

Boulton, M.G. and Williams, A. (1983). Health education in the general practice consultation: doctors' advice on diet, alcohol and smoking. *Health Education Journal*, 3, 57–63.

Boulton, M.G. and Williams, A. (1986). Health education and prevention in general practice – the views of GP trainees. *Health Education Journal*, 45, 79–83.

Bray, C. and Ward, C. (1986). *Ischaemic heart disease*. London: Update publications.

British Medical Journal (1952). Report of the General Practice Steering Committee: a college of general practitioners. *British Medical Journal*, 2, 1321.

Butler, J.R. and Calnan, M. (1987). *Too many patients? The economy of time and standards of care in general practice*. Aldershot: Gower Press.

Calnan, M. (1982). A review of government policies aimed at primary cancer prevention, in Alderson, M. (ed.) *Prevention of cancer*. London: Edward Arnold.

Calnan, M. (1984). The politics of health: the case of smoking control. *Journal of Social Policy*, 3, 279–96.

Calnan, M. (1987). *Health and illness; the lay perspective*. London: Tavistock.

Calnan, M. (1988a). Variations in the range of services provided by GPs. *Family Practice*, 5, 2, 94–104.

Calnan, M. (1988b). Images of general practice. *Social Science and Medicine*, 27, 6, 579–86.

Calnan, M. (1989). Control over health and patterns of health-related behaviour. *Social Science and Medicine*, 29, 2, 131–6.

Calnan, M. (1990). Food and health, in Cunningham, S. Burley, S. and McKeganey, N. *Readings in medical sociology*. London: Tavistock.

Calnan, M., Boulton, M. and Williams, A. (1987). The role of the general practitioner in health education: a critical appraisal, in Watt, A. and Rodmell, S. (eds) *The politics of health education*. London: Routledge & Kegan Paul.

Calnan, M. and Butler, J.R. (1988). The economy of time in general practice: an estimate of the influence of list size. *Social Science and Medicine*, 26, 4, 435–551.

Calnan, M. and Cant, S. (1990). The social organisation of food consumption. *Int J of Sociology and Social Policy*, 10, 2, 53–79.

Calnan, M. and Gabe, J. (1991). Recent developments in general practice: a sociological analysis, in Gabe, J., Calnan, M. and Bury, M. (eds) *The sociology of the Health Service*, London: Routledge.

Calnan, M. and Johnson, B. (1983). Influencing health behaviour: how significant is the GP? *Health Education Journal*, 43, 31–45.

Calnan, M. and Johnson, B. (1985). Health, health risks and inequalities: an exploratory study of women's perceptions. *Sociology of Health and Illness*, 7, 55–75.

Calnan, M. and Rutter, D.R. (1986). Do health beliefs predict health behaviour? *Social Science and Medicine*, 22, 673–8.

Calnan, M. and Williams, S. (1991). Style of life and the salience of health. *Sociology of Health and Illness*, (in press).

Calnan, S.E. (1989). Old people's perceptions of illness and old age. University of Kent: unpublished MPhil thesis.

Cameron, D. and Jones, I.G. (1985). An epidemiological and sociological analysis of the use of alcohol, tobacco and other drugs of solace. *Community Medicine*, 7, 18–29.

Cartwright, A. and Anderson, R. (1981). *General practice revisited: a second study of patients and their doctors*. London: Tavistock.

Charles, N. and Kerr, M. (1986a). Eating properly; the family and state benefit. *Sociology*, 20, 3, 412–29.

Charles, N. and Kerr, M. (1986b). Issues of responsibility and control in the feeding of families, in Rodmell, S. and Watt, A. (eds) *The politics of health education*. London: Routledge.

Charles, N. and Kerr, M. (1986c). Servers and providers: the distribution of food within the family. *Sociological Review*, 34, 1, 115–57.

Charles, N. and Kerr, M. (1987). Just the way it is: gender and age differences and family food consumption, in Brannen, J. and Wilson, G. (eds) *Give and take in families: studies in resource distribution*. Manchester: Allen & Unwin.

Cohen, D.R. (1984). Economic consequences of non-smoking generation. Health Economics Research Unit, University of Aberdeen. Discussion Paper 06184.

Cole-Hamilton, I. (1989). Review of food patterns amongst lower income groups in the UK. *Health Education Authority* (unpublished report).

Collins, M. (1987). *The sociology of sport and exercise in the UK*. London: The Coronary Prevention Group.

Consensus Conference (1985). Lowering blood cholesterol to prevent heart disease. *JAMA*, 253, ix–20.

Cook, D.G. (1986). Can we detect an effect of unemployment on cardiovascular morbidity or mortality? *Coronary Prevention Group*, 131–142, London.

Cook, D.G., Pocock, S.J., Shaper, A.G. and Kussick, S.J. (1986). Giving up smoking and the risk of heart attacks. *Lancet*, 11, 1376–9.

Corney, R. and Calnan, M. (1991). Job satisfaction and the new contract. *British Medical Journal*, (in press).

Cornwell, J. (1984). *Hard-earned lives*. London: Tavistock.

Coronary Prevention Group. (1989). *Background statistics on the prevalence of CHD*. London: Coronary Prevention Group.

Coronary Prevention Group. (1990). Coronary heart disease prevention in primary care: making it happen. Report of a Workshop, London: Wordworks.

Cowie, B. (1976). Cardiac perceptions of a heart attack. *Social Science and Medicine*, 10, 87–96.

Cox, H. (1984). Smoking, tobacco promotion and the voluntary agreements. *British Medical Journal*, 288, 303–5.

Cox, H. and Smith, R. (1984). Political approaches to smoking control; a comparative analysis. *Applied Economics*, 1, 17–25.

Crawford, R. (1984). A cultural account of 'health': control, release and the social body, in McKinlay, J. (ed.) *Issues in the political economy of health care*. London: Tavistock.

CSO (Central Statistical Office). (1989). *Social Trends 1988/89*. London:

HMSO.

Cutler, J.A., Neaton, J.D., Hulley, S.B., Kuller, L., Ogelsby, P. and Stamler, J. (1985). Coronary heart disease and all-cause mortality in the multiple risk factor intervention trial; subgroup findings and comparison with other trials. *Preventive Medicine*, 14, 293–311.

Davies, C. (1984). General practitioners and the pull of prevention. *Sociology of Health and Illness*, 6 (3), 267–84.

Davies, P. and Walsh, P. (1983). *Alcohol problems and alcohol control in Europe*. London: Croom Helm.

DHSS (Department of Health and Social Security). (1976). *Prevention and health: everybody's business*. London: HMSO.

DHSS (Department of Health and Social Security). (1978). *Eating for health*. London: HMSO.

DHSS (Department of Health and Social Security). (1981). *Drinking sensibly*. London: HMSO.

DHSS (Department of Health and Social Security). (1984). *Diet and cardiovascular disease*. London: HMSO.

DHSS (Department of Health and Social Security). (1989). *Working for patients*. London: HMSO.

DHSS/HEC (Department of Health and Social Security/Health Education Council). (1986). 'Look after your heart' campaign. Consultative document. *HEC*.

Department of Health and Welsh Office. (1989). *General practice in the NHS: a new contract*. London.

Doll, R. and Peto, R. (1976). Mortality in relation to smoking. *British Medical Journal*, 2, 1523–36.

Doyal, L. (1979). *The political economy of health*. London: Pluto Press.

D'Souza, M.F., Swan, A.V. and Shannon, D.J. (1976). A long-term controlled trial of screening for hypertension in general practice. *Lancet*, 1, 1228–31.

Duffy, J.C. and Plant, M.A. (1986). Scotland's liquor licensing changes: an assessment. *British Medical Journal*, 292, 36–9.

Elkan, W. (1988). Coronary heart disease: economic aspects of prevention. *Lipid Review*, 2, 6, 42–6.

Enthoven, A.H. (1985). *Reflections on the management of the National Health Service*. London: Nuffield Provincial Hospitals Trust.

Epstein, F.H. (1984). Lessons from falling coronary heart disease mortality in the US. *Postgraduate Medical Journal*, 60, 15–19.

Farquhar, J.W., Maccoby, N., Wood, P.D., Alexander, J.K., Breitrose, H., Brown, B.W., Haskell, I.V., McAlister, A.L., Meyer, A.J., Nash, J.D. and Stern, M.P. (1977). Community education for cardiovascular health. *Lancet*, 1, 1192–5.

Farrant, W. and Russell, J. (1987). *The politics of health information*. London: Institute of Education.

Fishbein, M. and Ajzen, I. (1975). *Attitude, intention and behavior: an introduction to theory and research*. Boston: Addison-Wesley.

Fleming, D. and Lawrence, M. (1981). An evaluation of recorded information about preventive measures in 38 practices. *Journal of the Royal College of General Practitioners*, 31, 615–20.

Forbes, J.F. (1988). Public policy and primary medical care in the UK:

an economic perspective on promoting health. *Family Practice*, 5, 4, 237–41.

Ford, A.S. and Ford, W.S. (1983). Health education and the primary care physician; the practitioner's perspective. *Soc Sci and Med*, 17, 1502–5.

Fowler, G. (1986). Does health education in general practice work? *Health Education Journal*, 45; 59–60.

Freidson, E. (1985). The reorganization of the medical profession. *Medical Care Review*, 42, 11, 11–35.

Fujii, E. (1980). The demand for cigarettes: further empirical evidence and its implications for public policy. *Applied Economics*, 12, 479–89.

Fullard, E., Fowler, G. and Gray, M. (1987). Promoting prevention in primary care: controlled trial of low technology, low cost approach. *British Medical Journal*, 294, 1080–2.

General Medical Services Committee. (1983). *General practice: a British success*. London: BMA.

Godfrey, C. (1986). Government policy, advertising and tobacco consumption in the UK. A critical review of the literature. *B.J. Addiction*, 81, 339–46.

Godfrey, C. and Maynard, A. (1988). Economic aspects of tobacco use and taxation policy. *British Medical Journal*, 297, 339–43.

Goldmann, L. and Cook, E.F. (1984). The decline in IHD mortality rates: an analysis of the comparative effects of medical intervention and changes in lifestyle. *Ann Intern Med*, 101, 825–36.

Gotto, A.M. (1988). Co-existent hypercholesterolaemia and hypertension in CHD risk: clinical aspects and considerations, *Lipid Review*, 2, 3, 17–22.

Grace, J. (1983). Screening in general practice: implications for cost and extra work. *British Medical Journal*, 287, 589–90.

Graham, H. (1979). Prevention and health: every mother's business: a comment on child health policies in the 1970s, in Harris, D. (ed.) *The sociology of the family: new directions for Britain*. Sociological Review Monographs 18, Keele: University of Keele.

Graham, H. (1987). Being poor, in Brannen, J. and Wilson, G. (eds) *Give and take in families: studies of resource distribution*. London: Allen & Unwin.

Graham, H. (1989). Women and smoking in the UK: the implications for health promotion. *Health Promotion*, 3, 4, 371–81.

Gregory, J., Foster, K., Tyler, H. and Wiseman, M. (1990). *The dietary and nutritional survey of British adults*. London: HMSO.

Haigh-Smith, C. and Armstrong, D. (1989). Comparison of criteria derived by government and patients for evaluating general practitioner services. *British Medical Journal*, 299, 494–6.

HEC (Health Education Council). (1984). *The prevention of coronary heart disease: the Canterbury Report*. London: Pitman Publishing Co.

HEC (Health Education Council). (1985). *Eating for a healthier heart*. London: JACNE.

Heartbeat Wales. (1987). Pulse of Wales. Report no 7, Heartbeat Wales, 24 Park Place, Cardiff, CF1 3BA.

Helman, C. (1987). Heart disease and the cultural construction of time: the type A behaviour pattern as a Western culture-bound syndrome. *Social Science and Medicine*, 25, 9, 969–79.

Hjermann, I. (1983). A randomised primary preventive trial in coronary heart disease: the Oslo study. *Preventive Medicine*, 12, 1, 181–4.

HMSO. (1989). *Public Accounts Committee: report on CHD*. London: HMSO.

Honigsbaum, F. (1985). Reconstruction of general practice: the failure of reform. *British Medical Journal*, 290, 823–6.

Horder, J., Bosanquet, N. and Stocking, B. (1986). Ways of influencing the behaviour of general practitioners. *J of Royal College of General Practitioners*, 36, 517–21.

Hunt, S. and Mcleod, M. (1987). Health and behavioural change: some lay perspectives. *Community Medicine*, 9, 1, 68–76.

Intersalt Co-operative Research Group. (1989). Intersalt: an international study of electrolyte excretion and blood pressure. *British Medical Journal*, 297, 319–28.

Jacobsen, B. (1981). *The ladykillers: why smoking is a feminist issue*. London: Pluto Press.

Jamrozik, K. and Fowler, G. (1982). Anti-smoking education in Oxfordshire general practices. *J of the Royal College of General Practitioners*, 32, 1179–83.

Janz, N. and Becker, M. (1984). The health belief model: a decade later. *Health Educ Quarterly*, 11, 1–47.

Jefferys, M. and Sachs, H. (1983). *Rethinking general practice: dilemmas in primary medical care*. London: Tavistock.

Johnston, D.W., Cook, D.G. and Shaper, A.G. (1987). Type A behaviour and ischaemic heart disease in middle aged British men. *British Medical Journal*, 295, 86–9

Jones, A., Davies, D.H., Dove, J.R., Collinson, M.A. and Brown, P.M. (1988). Identification and treatment of risk factors for coronary heart disease in general practice: a possible screening model. *British Medical Journal*, 296, 1711–15.

Jones, D. (1986). Heart disease mortality following widowhood: some results from the OPCS longitudinal study. *Coronary Prevention Group*, 77–102. London.

Kannell, W.B. (1975). Risk of blood pressure in cardiovascular disease: the Framingham study. *Angiol*, 26, 1–14.

Karasek, R.A. (1979). Job demands, job decision latitude and mental strain: implications for job redesign. *Admin Sci Qtrly*, 24, 285–307.

Keys, A., Aravnis, C., Van Buchem, F.S.P., Blackburn, H., Bouzina, R., Djordjevic, B.S., Dontas, S., Fidinza, F., Carvoneu, M.J., Kimura, N., Menotti, A., Nedeljkovic, S., Puddu, V., Punsar, S. and Taylor H.L. (1981). The diet and all-cause death rate in the seven countries study. *Lancet*, 2, 58–61.

Kiely, B.G. and McPherson, I.G. (1986). Stress self-help packages in primary care: a controlled trial evaluation. *J of the Royal College of General Practitioners*, 36, 307–9.

King's Fund. (1985). *Coronary artery bypass surgery: Consensus statement*. London.

King's Fund. (1989). *Consensus Conference on Cholesterol*. London.

Labonté, R. and Penfold, S. (1981). Canadian perspectives in health promotion: a critique. *Health Education*, April, 4–8.

Langlie, J.K. (1979). Interrelationships among preventive health behaviours: a test of competing hypotheses. *Public Health Rep*, 94, 216–20.

Lempo, K. and Vertio, H. (1986). Smoking control in Finland: as case study in policy formulation and implementation. *Health Promotion*, 1, 1, 5–16.

Leu, R.E. and Schaub, T. (1983). Does smoking increase medical care expenditure? *Soc Sci and Med*, 17, 223, 1907–14.

Lewis, B., Mann, J.I. and Mancini, M. (1986). Reducing the risk of CHD in individuals and in the population. *Lancet*, 1, 956–8.

Lichtenstein, M.J., Shipley, M.J. and Rose, G. (1985). Systolic and diastolic blood pressures as predictors of coronary heart disease mortality in the Whitehall study. *British Medical Journal*, 291, 243–5.

Lipid Research Clinic's Program. (1984). The Lipid Research Clinic's coronary primary prevention trial results 1. Reduction in incidence of CHD. *JAMA*, 252, 351–64.

McCormick, J. and Skrabanek, P. (1988). Coronary heart disease is not preventable by population interventions. *Lancet*, 839–41.

McGuiness, T. and Cowling, K.C. (1975). Advertising and the aggregate demand for cigarettes. *European Economic Review*, 6, 311–28.

McKenzie, J. (1988). Positive move on heart disease. *Health Education Journal*, 47, 1, 36–7.

McWhinney, I. (1964). *The early signs of illness*. London: Pitman Publishing Co.

Madge, N. and Marmot, M. (1987). Psychosocial factors and health. *Quarterly J of Soc Affairs*, 3, 121, 81–134.

MAFF (Ministry of Agriculture, Fisheries and Food). (1987). *Household consumption and expenditure: annual reports of the National Food Survey Committee*. London: HMSO.

MAFF (Ministry of Agriculture, Fisheries and Food). (1987/8). *Guidelines on nutrition labelling*. London: HMSO.

Mann, J.L. (1987). Clinical trials of cholesterol lowering. *Lipid Review*, 1, 4, 25–33.

Mann, J.L. (1989). Population strategies for the prevention of coronary heart disease. *Lipid Review*, 2, 7, 49–54.

Mann, J.L., Lewis, B., Shepherd, J., Winder, A.F., Fenster, S., Rose, L. and Morgan, B. (1988). Blood lipid concentrations and other cardiovascular risk factors: distribution, prevalence and detection in Britain. *British Medical Journal*, 296, 1702–6.

Markowe, H.L.J., Marmot, M.G., Shipley M.J., Bulpitt, C.J., Meade, T.W., Stirling, Y., Vickers, M.V. and Semmence, A. (1985). Fibrinogen: a possible link between social class and coronary heart disease. *British Medical Journal*, 291, 1312–14.

Marmot, M. (1984). Life style and national and international trends in coronary heart disease mortality. *Postgraduate Medical Journal*, 60, 3–8.

Marmot, M. (1986). *Can stress cause CHD*? London: Coronary Prevention Group.

Marmot, M. and McDowall, M.E. (1986). Mortality decline and widening social inequalities. *Lancet*, ii, 274–6.

Marmot, M., Shipley, M.J. and Rose, G. (1984). Inequalities in death – specific explanations of a general pattern. *Lancet*, 1, 1003–7.

Marmot, M. and Theorell, T. (1988). Social class and cardiovascular disease: the contribution of work. *Int J of Health Services*, 18, 4, 659–74.

Marmot, M. and Winkelstein, W. (1975). Epidemiologic observation on intervention trials for prevention of CHD. *American Journal of Epidemiology*, 101, 177–81.

Marsh, A. (1984). Smoking: habit or choice? *Population Trends*, 37, 14–20.

Marsh, A. and Matheson, J. (1983). *Smoking attitudes and behaviour*. London: HMSO.

Martin, M.J., Hulley, S.B., Browner, W.S., Kuller, L.H. and Wentworth, D.H. (1986). Serum cholesterol, blood pressure and mortality. *Lancet*, ii, 933–6.

Maynard, A. (1984). Reassessing NHS evaluation could prove a 'blooming' success. *Health and Social Services Journal*, 13 December, 1467.

Maynard, A. (1986). Economic aspects of addiction policy. *Health Promotion*, 1, 1, 61–72.

Mechanic, D. (1970). Practice orientations among general medical practitioners in England and Wales. *Med Care*, viii, 15–25.

Milio, N. (1981). Promoting health through structural change: analysis of the ongoing implementation of Norway's farm food nutrition policy. *Social Science and Medicine*, 13, 121–34.

Milio, N. (1985). Health policy and the emerging tobacco reality. *Social Science and Medicine*, 21, 603–13.

Milio, N. (1989). Nutrition and health: patterns and policy perspectives in food rich countries. *Social Science and Medicine*, 29, 3, 413–24.

Morgan, M., Heller, R. and Swedlow, A. (1989). Changes in diet and coronary heart disease mortality among social classes in Great Britain. *J. of Epid and Comm Health*, 43, 102–16.

Morrell, D.C. (1989). The new general practitioner contract in The NHS Review – what it means. *British Medical Journal*, 23, London.

Morris, J. (1986). Exercise: why bother? *Times Health Supplement*, September, 5–6.

Morris, J., Everitt, M.G., Pollard, R., Chave, S.P.W. and Semmence, A.M. (1980). Vigorous exercise in leisure-time, protection against CHD. *Lancet*, 2, 1207–10.

MRC (Medical Research Council Working Party). (1985). MRC trial of treatment of mild hypertension: principal results. *Lancet*, 291, 97–104.

National Audit Office. (1989). *National Health Service: coronary heart disease*. London: HMSO.

National Forum for Coronary Heart Disease Prevention. (1988). *Coronary heart disease prevention: action in the UK 1984–1987*. London: Health Education Authority.

Neaton, J.D., Kuller, L.H., Wentworth, D. and Borhani, N.D. (1984). Total and cardiovascular mortality in relation to cigarette smoking, serum cholesterol concentration, and diastolic blood pressure among black and white males followed up for five years. *American Heart Journal*, 108, 759–69.

Neutze, J.M. and White, H.D. (1987). What contribution has cardiac surgery made to the decline in mortality from CHD? *British Medical Journal*, 294, 405–8.

Oliver, M.C. (1985). Strategies for preventing and screening for CHD. *British Heart Journal*, 54, 1–5.

OPCS (Office of Population Censuses and Surveys). (1986). *Occupational mortality. Decennial supplement*. London: HMSO.

OPCS (Office of Population Censuses and Surveys). (1986). *General household survey, 1984*. London: HMSO.

OPCS (Office of Population Censuses and Surveys). (1988). Monitor DH2 8813. London: HMSO

Open University. (1985a). *Caring for health, dilemmas and prospects.* Milton Keynes: Open University Press.

Open University (1985b). *The biology of health and disease*. Milton Keynes: Open University Press.

Paffenburger, R.S., Wing, A.L. and Hyde, R.T. (1978). Physical activity as an index of heart attack risk in college alumni. *American Journal of Epidemiology*, 108, 161–75.

Pearson, T.A. (1988). *Determinants of coronary heart disease mortality*. Oxford: Oxford University Press.

Pendleton, D. and Bochner, S. (1980). The communication of medical information in general practice consultations and function of patients 'social class'. *Social Science and Medicine*, 14A, 664–73.

Peto, J. (1974). Price and consumption of cigarettes and a case of intervention. *British Journal of Preventative and Social Medicine*, 28, 241–5.

Pickard, B. (1986). Dairy products and red meat: villains or victims?, in Anderson, D. *A diet of reason*. London: Social Affairs Unit.

Pill, R. and Parry, O. (1989). Making changes – women, food and families. *Health Education Journal*, 48, 2, 51–4.

Pill, R. and Stott, N. (1982). Concepts of illness causality and responsibility: some preliminary data from a sample working class mothers. *Social Science and Medicine*, 16, 143–9.

Pisa, Z. and Uemura, K. (1982). Trends of mortality for ischaemic heart disease and other cardiovascular disease in 27 countries 1968–77. *World Health Statistics Quarterly*, 35, 11–16.

Player, D. (1986). The big killer. *World Health*, 12 June, 4–5.

Pocock, S.J., Cook, D.G., Shaper, A.G., Phillips, A.N. and Walker, M. (1987). Social class differences in ischaemic heart disease in British men. Lancet, ii, 197–201.

Pollock, K. (1988). On the nature of social stress: production of a modern mythology. *Social Science and Medicine*, 26, 3, 381–91.

Puska, P., Nissinen, A., Salanen, J.T. and Toumilchto, J. (1983). Ten years of the North Karelia Project: results with community-based prevention of CHD. *Scandinavian Journal of Social Medicine*, 11, 65–8.

Raw, M. (1989). Tobacco and Europe: Britain against the rest. *British Medical Journal*, 298, 140.

Rayner, M. (1989) The truth about the British diet. *New Scientist*, 22 July, 44–7.

RCGP (Royal College of General Practitioners). (1959). *Preventive health care in general practice*. Archives of the Royal College of General Practitioners.

RCGP (Royal College of General Practitioners). (1981a). *Health and prevention in primary care: report from general practice 18*. London:

Royal College of General Practitioners.

RCGP (Royal College of General Practitioners). (1981b). *Prevention of arterial disease in general practice: report from general practice 19*. London: Royal College of General Practitioners.

RCGP (Royal College of General Practitioners). (1981c). *Prevention of psychiatric disorders in general practice: report from general practice 20*. London: Royal College of General Practitioners.

RCGP (Royal College of General Practitioners). (1981d). *Family planning – an exercise in preventive medicine: report from general practice 21*. London: Royal College of General Practitioners.

RCGP (Royal College of General Practitioners). (1982). *Healthier children – thinking prevention: report from general practice 22*. London: Royal College of General Practitioners.

Reid, D.D., Hamilton, P.J.S., McCartney, P., Rose, G., Jarrett, R.J. and Keen, H. (1976). Smoking and other risk factors for CHD in British civil servants. *Lancet*, ii, 979–84.

Ritchie, L.D. and Currie, A.M. (1983). Blood pressure recording by GPs in north east Scotland. *British Medical Journal*, 286, 107–9.

Roberts, J. (1986). Code busting by the tobacco companies. North West Regional Health Authority.

Robinson, D., Maynard, A. and Chester, R. (eds). (1989). *Controlling legal addictions*. London: Macmillan.

Robinson, R. (1989). New health care market in *The NHS Review* – what it means. *British Medical Journal*, 298, 437–9.

Robson, J., Black, Sir D., Clark, D.H., Curran, R.O., Feroze, R.M., Gillingham, F.J., Horder, J., Laws, J.W., Strong, J.A. and Taylor, P.J. (1982). Sponsorship of sport by tobacco companies. *British Medical Journal*, 284, 395–6.

Roemer, R. (1982). *Legislative action to combat the world smoking epidemic*. Geneva: World Health Organisation.

Rose, G. (1975). The contribution of intensive coronary care. *British Journal of Preventative Social Medicine*, 29, 147–50.

Rose, G. (1981). Strategy of prevention: lessons from cardiovascular disease. *British Medical Journal*, 282, 1817–908.

Rose, G., Hamilton, P.J.S., Golwell, L. and Shipley, M.J. (1982). A randomised controlled trial of anti-smoking advice. *Journal of Epidemiology and Community Health*, 36, 102–8.

Rose, G. and Marmot, M. (1981). Social class and CHD. *British Heart Journal*, 145, 13–19.

Royal College of Physicians. (1962). *Smoking and health*. London: Pitman Publishing Co.

Royal College of Physicians. (1971). *Smoking and health now*. London: Pitman Publishing Co.

Royal College of Physicians. (1977). *Smoking or health*. London: Pitman Publishing Co.

Royal College of Physicians. (1983a). *Health and smoking*. London: Pitman Publishing Co.

Royal College of Physicians. (1983b). *Obesity*. London: Pitman Publishing Co.

Royston/Wardieburn Project. (1986). *Report*. Edinburgh: Royston/Wardieburn Community Health Project.

Russell, J. (1986). *Coronary heart disease and Asians in Britain*. London: Coronary Prevention Group.

Russell, L.D. (1986). *Is prevention better than cure*? Washington: Brookings Institute.

Russell, M.A.H. (1973). Changes in cigarette price and consumption by men in Britain, 1946–71. *British Journal of Preventative Medicine*, 27, 1–7.

Russell, M.A.H., Stapleton, J., Hajek, P., Jackson, P. and Belcher, M. (1987). District programme to reduce smoking: effect of clinic supported brief intervention by general practitioners. *British Medical Journal*, 295, 1240–4.

Russell, M.A.H., Stapleton, J., Hajek, P., Jackson, P. and Belcher, M. (1988). District programme to reduce smoking: can sustained intervention by general practitioners affect prevalence? *J of Epid and Comm Health*, 42, 111–15.

Sanderson, M. and Winkler, J.T. (1983). Strategies for implementing NACNE recommendations. *Lancet*, 2, 1353–4.

Sanderson, M. and Winkler, J.T. (1990). *Towards a Sugarus policy; a model for food and health*. London: Smith-Gordon.

Saunders, B. and Allsop, S. (1983). Giving up addictions. Paisley College of Technology, mimeo.

Secretaries of State for Health Services. (1987). *Promoting better health*. London: HMSO.

Shaper, A.G. (1986). Diet and heart disease. Postgraduate Doctor, Middle East, 674, 9, 11, 614–22.

Shaper, A.G., Cook, D.G., Walker, M. and Macfarlane, P.W. (1984a). Prevalence of ischaemic heart disease in middle-aged British men. *British Heart Journal*, 51, 595–605.

Shaper, A.G., Cook, D.G., Walker, M. and Macfarlane, P.W. (1984b). Recall of diagnosis by men with ischaemic heart disease. *British Heart Journal*, 51, 606–11.

Shaper, A.G., and Pocock, S.J., (1985). British blood cholesterol values and the American Consensus. *British Medical Journal*, 291, 480–1.

Shaper, A.G. Pocock, S.J. Walker, M., Phillips, A.W., Whitehead, T.P. and Macfarlane, P.W. (1985). Risk factors for ischaemic heart disease: the prospective phase of the British Regional Heart Study. *Journal of Epidemiology and Community Health*, 39, 197–209.

Shaper, A.G., Pocock, S.T., Phillips, A.W. and Walker, M. (1986). Identifying men at high risk of heart attacks: strategy for use in general practice. *British Medical Journal*, 193, 474–9.

Sharp, I. and Rayner, M. (1990). Cholesterol testing with desk-top machines. *Lancet*, 335, 55.

Smith, A. (1987). Qualms about QALYs. *Lancet*, 1134–6.

Smith, W.C.S., Crombie, I.K., Tavendale, R.T., Galland, S.K. and Tunstall-Pedoe, H.D. (1988). Urinary electrolyte excretion, alcohol consumption and blood pressure in the Scottish heart health study. *British Medical Journal*, 297, 329–30.

Smith, W.C.S., Kenicer, M.B., Maryon–Davis, A., Evans, A.E., Harnell, J. (1989). Blood cholesterol: is population screening warranted in the UK? *Lancet*, 18 Feb, 372–3.

St George, D.P. (1983). Is coronary heart disease caused by an environmentally induced chronic metabolic imbalance? *Medical Hypotheses*, 12, 283–96.

Stoate, H.G. (1989). Can health screening damage your health? *J of Royal College of General Practitioners*, 39, 193–5.

Stott, N. and Davis, R. (1979) The exceptional potential in each primary care consultation. *J of Royal College of General Practitioners*, 19, 201–5.

Sutton, S. (1987). Socio-psychological approaches to understanding addictive behaviours: attitude-behaviour and decision making models. *British Journal of Addiction*, 82, 355–73.

Sutton, S. (1989). Smoking attitudes and behaviour: applications of Fishbein and Ajzen's theory of reasoned action to predicting and understanding smoking decisions, in Ney, T. and Gale, A. (eds) *Smoking and human behaviour*. Chichester: Wiley.

Swales, J.D. (1981). *Clinical hypertension*. London: Chapman & Hall.

Taylor, P. (1984). *Smoke ring: the politics of tobacco*. London: Bodley Head.

Thelle, D.S., Shaper, A.G., Whitehead, T.P., Bullock, D.G., Ashby, D. and Patel, S. (1983). Blood lipids in middle aged men. *British Heart Journal*, 149, 205–13.

Thom, T.J., Epstein, F.H., Feldman, J.J. and Leaverton, P.E. (1985). Trends in total mortality and morbidity from heart disease in 26 countries from 1950–1970. *International Journal of Epidemiology*, 14, 510–20.

Townsend, J. (1987). Economics and health consequences of smoking, in Williams, A. (ed.) *Health and economics*. London: Macmillan.

Townsend, P., and Davidson, N. (1982). *Inequalities in health*. London: Penguin.

Townsend, P., Davidson, N. and Whitehead, M. (1988). *Inequalities in health*. London: Penguin.

Tracey, R. (1987). Opening address: Exercise Heart Health Conference. London: The Coronary Prevention Group.

Truswell, A.S. (1985a). Reducing the risk of CHD. *British Medical Journal*, 291, 34–7.

Truswell, A.S. (1985b). Diet and hypertension. *British Medical Journal*, 291, 125–7.

Tuckett, D., Boulton, M., Olson, C. and Williams, A. (1985). *Meetings between experts*. London: Tavistock.

Tunstall-Pedoe, H. (1989). Who is for cholesterol testing? *British Medical Journal*, 298, 1593–4.

Tunstall-Pedoe, H., Smith, W.L.S. and Tavendale, R. (1989). How-often-that-high graphs of serum cholesterol, *Lancet*, i, 540–2.

US National Committee on Detection, Evaluation and Treatment of High Blood Pressure. (1986). 1984 report. *J LA State Med-Soc*, 138, 51–64.

Vines, G. (1989). Diet, drugs and heart disease. *New Scientist*, 25 February, 44–9.

Wadsworth, M.E.J., Cripps, H.A., Midwinter, R.E. and Culley, J.R.T. (1985). Blood pressure in a national birth cohort at the age of 36 related to social and familial factors, smoking and body mass. *British Medical Journal*, 291, 1534–9.

Walker, C. (1984). The national diet. *Postgraduate Medical Journal*, 160, 26–33.

Walker, C. and Cannon, G. (1984). *The food scandal*. London: Century Publishing.

Wallace, P.G., Brennan, P.J. and Haines, A.P. (1987). Are general practitioners doing enough to promote healthy lifestyles? *British Medical Journal*, 294, 940–2.

Wallston, K., Wallston, B. and De Veilra, R. (1978). Development of the multi-dimensional health locus of control (MHLC) scales. *Health Educ Monographs* 6, 160–73.

Wasfie, T.J. and Brown, A. (1981). Coronary grafting: a sound investment. *The Practitioner*, 225, 739–44.

Watt, A. (1984). Community health initiatives: clarifying the complexity. Paper given at conference on Community Health Initiatives, King's Fund Centre, London, 14 June.

Wheatley, D. (1984). Surgical prospects. Paper given at Consensus Development Conference on CABG. London: King's Fund.

Wells, N. (1982). *Coronary heart disease: scope for prevention*. London: Office of Health Economics.

Wells, N. (1987). *Coronary heart disease: the need for action, No. 86*. London: Office of Health Economics.

Wheelock, V. (1986). *The food revolution*. Marlow: Chalcombe Publications.

Wheelock, V. and Fallows, S. (1985). *Implications of the COMA report on diet and cardiovascular disease for British agriculture food policy research*. Bradford: University of Bradford.

WHO (World Health Organisation). (1982). Technical report: prevention of CHD, series no. 618. Geneva: WHO.

WHO (World Health Organisation). (1983). Primary prevention of essential hypertension. Report of a scientific group. Geneva: WHO.

WHO (World Health Organisation). (1984). Expert committee on community prevention and control of CHD. Copenhagen: WHO.

WHO (World Health Organisation). (1986). Community prevention and control of cardiovascular diseases. Report of a WHO expert committee, technical report no. 732. Copenhagen: WHO.

Wilkin, D., Hallam, L., Leavey, R. and Metcalfe, D. (1987). *Anatomy of urban general practice*. London: Tavistock.

Wilkinson, J. (1986). *Tobacco: the facts behind the smokescreen*. London: Penguin.

Williams, A. (1987). Screening for risk of CHD: is it a wise use of resources?, in Oliver, M., Ashley-Miller, M. and Wood, D. (eds) *Screening for risk of coronary heart disease*. Chichester: Wiley.

Williams, S. and Calnan, M. (1991). Assessing consumer satisfaction with primary care. In press.

Wilson, G. (1989). Diet and health. *Journal of Social Policy*, 18. 167–85.

Winkelstein, W. and Marmot, M. (1981). Primary prevention of ischaemic heart disease: evaluation of community interventions. *Annual Review of Public Health*, 2, 253–60.

Winkler, J. (1987). Food is a political issue. *The Health Service Journal*, 6 August, 910.

Wrench, J.G. and Irvine, R.C. (1984). Coronary heart disease: an account of a preventative clinic in general practice. *Journal of the Royal College of General Practitioners*, 34, 477–81.

Name index

Subject index